Psychopathology Explains Endocrino-Immunological Responses

(The relationship between the brain, spirit and defense system against diseases)

Hajime Jozuka, M.D.
Belong to "Jozuka Mental Clinic & JMC Stress Medical Institute
Address:
4-38, Takahatacho, Nishio, Aichi, Japan
zip code: 445-0064
Mail address: hajime_j@icloud.com

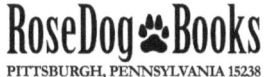

The contents of this work, including, but not limited to, the accuracy of events, people, and places depicted; opinions expressed; permission to use previously published materials included; and any advice given or actions advocated are solely the responsibility of the author, who assumes all liability for said work and indemnifies the publisher against any claims stemming from publication of the work.

All Rights Reserved
Copyright © 2016 by Hajime Jozuka, M.D.

No part of this book may be reproduced or transmitted, downloaded, distributed, reverse engineered, or stored in or introduced into any information storage and retrieval system, in any form or by any means, including photocopying and recording, whether electronic or mechanical, now known or hereinafter invented without permission in writing from the publisher.

RoseDog Books
585 Alpha Drive
Suite 103
Pittsburgh, PA 15238
Visit our website at *www.rosedogbookstore.com*

ISBN: 978-1-4809-7273-5
eISBN 978-1-4809-7296-4

For Dr. Ryosuke Jozuka

Preface for the III-rd. Edition

It is the great pleasure of this author to have published articles contained in this medical book, including articles on the relationship between psychopathology, neurology, endocrinology and immunology, called "Psycho-neuro-endocrino-immuno-pathology." This word seems too long to be easily understood. However, the word is appropriate to serve as the fundamental ideation of this book. The author acknowledges that this situation is the first to be published as a monograph studied by a psychiatrist. The importance of studying this relationship in medical areas has been clarified by not only several medical and social researchers but also common people. As a result, thus, it was necessary to convey these ideas through the publication of this book, the time was reached this situation. The living creatures will be able to continue to live with the in establishment of defense mechanisms and offensive mechanisms. Therefore Regarding to this establishment, human beings will continue to live uncharged. For example, humans will suffer from diabetes mellitus when the instinct against sweet food including alcohol is continuously increased. However, as defense mechanisms increase, humans will suffer from autoimmune diseases or malignant neoplasms because the mechanisms of both diseases are considered a type of defense in that same human body and mind. In autoimmune diseases, different components of the same individual fight against one another. Furthermore, a malignant neoplasm is created inside a host, and this same neoplasm will attempt to kill this host. These situations pique our curiosity although these diseases occur in both humans and other creatures.

At the time of the publication of this book, diseases must be considered in their entirety to account for the appearance of these diseases. Let us consider the entire disease in the whole creature to appear due to a given course and motivation, including both conscious and unconscious factors.

Thus, the entire processes and mechanisms responsible for diseases must be clarified in psychopathology. The author does not consider psychopathology to be the complete ideation; rather, it is an incomplete idea. However, psychopathology is the foundation in which humans attempt to understand various organic situations and studies.

Therefore, when comprehensive medical studies are performed, therapists must be concerned with the relationship between clients and therapists in "psycho-neuro-endocrino-immuno-pathology." Naturally, no answer will be determined solely by cognitive science, in which the therapist does not have to worry about the relationship between himself/herself and the client.

For example, therapists must be concerned with the relationship between clients and therapists when providing psychotherapeutic treatment. Cognitive behavioral therapy is never considered an exact psychotherapy, although some psychiatrists in developing societies maintain that cognitive science is the only fundamental ideation in psychiatry. Unfortunately, such scientific persons do not consider or notice the existence of the human spirit and the spiritual human relationship in psychotherapy.

The author has invited various psychotherapists to discuss the types of therapy necessary and how to establish the relationship between clients and therapists. At last, he discovered a psychotherapeutic approach based on the existential philosophy of Heidegger, M. Heidegger's fundamental philosophy will be applied to some treatment methods in this book. Many of the results and data reported in these articles occurred only accidently and were not expected in advance. Any data in this book will be not conclusive but must be extrapolated on according to the development of all areas of science.

This is only a preliminary study in these areas; thus, please inform the author if more results develop in these areas.

The author and his fellows await the discovery of new results. Please continue further studies in this area without hesitation.

At last, because some of the fellows passed away several years ago, they will never know of this publication issued by a large publishing company. However, the author will inform them within several years.

Sincerely,
Hajime Jozuka, M.D.

The Author's Profile

- 1948 Born in Takaoka City, Japan
- 1973 Graduated Faculty of Medicine, Kanazawa National University
- 1973 Research Assistant at the Psychiatric Institute, Nagoya City University
- 1975 Chief of Psychiatry at Hamamatsu Mikatagahara Hospital
- 1979 Chief of Psychiatry at Toyohashi National Hospital
- 1979 Lecturer at Toyohashi Nursing College
- 1989 Director of Psychiatry at the Health Administration Center at Nippon Telephone and Telegram
- 1994 President of Jozuka Mental Clinic
- 1994 President of JMC Stress Medical Institute

Specialties:
- Psychoneuroimmunopathology, Sexology, Industrial Medicine, Pediatric Psychiatry, and Allergology

Official Posts:
- Japan Psychosomatic Medical Association:
- Directing Doctor of Psychosomatic Medicine
- Psychiatric Doctor
- Trustee

- Hekinan Kindergarten:
- Trustee

Published Books:
- Psychoneuroimmunopathology, Maruzen Japan, 2000
- Introduction to Psychoneuroimmunopathology and Clinical Practice, Bibliobooks, Israel (English language), 2004
- Personality Disorders, San-ichi Shobo, Tokyo, Japan, 2004
- Sexology, San-ichi Shobo, Tokyo, Japan, 2005
- From Conception to Adolescence, Bibliobooks, Israel (English language), 2006
- Love Manual, Japan Literary Company, 2006
- How to Fall in Love, Bibliobooks, Israel (English language), 2007
- The Book to Read Before Becoming a Medical Doctor, San-ichi Shobo, Tokyo, Japan, 2007
- The Snakepit, A Memoir of a Young Psychiatrist, Bibliobooks, Israel (English language), 2008

Preface

It is with great pleasure that I introduce psychoneuroimmunopathology (PNIP) in the context of medical research for the first time. I would like to describe how PNIP was established based on the progress of our studies.

PNIP is the most complete method of treating illness. It is a method based on the fundamental existential philosophy of the medical world. Furthermore, it is significant that the establishment of PNIP was based on Daseinsanalysis, which was developed based on Freud, Heidegger, von Weizsaecker, Binswanger, Boss, and Kimura. Daseinsanalysis is a psychopathological approach. It is defined, in part, as an "awareness of being" by the patient. It incorporates the idea that the therapist and patient should fight together against the disease—that they should observe the disease from the same perspective and fight against it with the same effort. Boss established his Daseinsanalysis Institute and conducted many studies that developed and refined this technique.

PNIP was not established to bring back the dead but to bring back the living—from terminal illness to life. The so-called top specialists usually inform terminal patients that they do not have long to live. However, many such patients would live and recover their health if they received even a little support or a certain type of help from their doctors. Human beings suffer from a weakness that allows them to resign themselves to death, although they may not die if they receive even the slightest amount of help.

Psychoneuroimmunopathology (PNIP) can provide this help.

PNIP has been developed over more than thirty years through an accumulation of studies and much experimentation. Furthermore, the exact method was refined by the suggestions of many psychopathologists and immunologists, and I gratefully acknowledge the contributions of Professor Bin Kimura, Professor Hisao Nakai, and Professor Medard Boss for the German psychopathology; Professor Osamu Nishikaze and Professor Baulieu for the neuroendocrinology; and Professor Mitsuo Yokoyama and Professor Shunsuke Migita for the experimental immunology.

PNIP began as an unlikely clinical experiment. Through our studies and research, however, it has developed into a methodology that saves lives.

PNIP fundamentally differs from psychoneuroimmunology (PNI), but they have been based on common studies. PNIP has been used mainly to treat so-called incurable diseases whereas PNI has remained more limited.

Because PNIP is based on traditional German psychopathology, it follows that treatment methods would involve the analysis of deep emotions and the life histories of clients.

Because PNIP was born of psychopathology, it has been shown to be an appropriate and effective method for treating incurable diseases. PNI, by contrast, was born of the study of human behavior; thus, it cannot be used to effectively treat incurable diseases.

The research in this monograph will show how PNIP has been used to treat incurable diseases based on the history of precise evidence. Of course, there will be ongoing studies of PNIP as long as life-threatening disease exists.

Medical Background of the Study

Studies of PNIP were initiated through the discovery in 1979 of the Bence-Jones protein in the urine of persons who had schizoaffective disorder. Although some research was available on the relationship between some immunoglobulins and schizophrenia, discussions and results were confusing until that time.

The following is my first article on this subject:

"Case of Schizoaffective Disorders Showing a Bence-Jones Protein in Urine During Acute Stage" *Jozuka, H.: Journal of Psychiatry 1979*

Introduction

It has been believed that a Bence-Jones protein is found in the urine of patients suffering from long-term multiple myeloma. It should be noted that all studies of Bence-Jones proteins have involved a multiple myeloma or malignant tumors of the bone marrow. Thus, many studies have examined the relationship between the immunological roles of Bence-Jones proteins and bone marrow tumors. Such studies have never been applied to psychiatric clients in the form of a psychosomatic study. We conducted a study to discover whether the Bence-Jones protein is present in the urine of people suffering from psychosis. Some very interesting findings resulted from this study.

Subjects and Methods
Subjects
Of the 150 clients who received consultation at our department of psychiatry in the six months between April 20 and October 30, 1979, there were 64 whose urine showed the Bence-Jones protein two or more times in quantitative testing.

Quantitative testing for the Bence-Jones protein was used for these psychiatric clients for the following reasons:

The Bence-Jones protein has been believed to be present in the urine of clients suffering only from malignant myeloma.

Because the brains of people suffering from psychiatric disorders have shown abnormal changes, it was suspected that brain phenomena affect unusual changes in biological levels.

The discovery of the Bence-Jones protein in the urine of a psychiatric client indicated a possible relationship between brain phenomena and malignant neoplasms.

Quantitative testing for the Bence-Jones protein is easier than testing with other immunological parameters. In addition, there is a short lag time between testing and results.

Methodology of Quantitative Testing:
Putnam Method: Fresh urine from the client (4.0 ml) is added to 1.0 ml of 2 M (pH 4.9) acetic acid buffer solution and heated in a warm bath (56 degrees centigrade) for 15 minutes. Those specimens displaying precipitation are regarded as positive. The Harrison Method (described below) is used for further confirmation.

Harrison Method: Twenty-five milliliters of fresh urine is filtered until clear and is confirmed positive by the sulfosalicylic method. Twenty milliliters of urine is determined to be litmus neutral or weakly acidic with 33 % (V/V) acetic acid. Five milliliters of urine is placed into each of three test tubes: (1) one drop of 33 % acetic acid is added to first tube; (2) two drops of 33 % acetic acid are added to the second tube; (3) nothing is added to the third tube. A beaker containing cold water is placed on an electric heater; a thermometer is placed into the water, and then the three test tubes described above are placed into the water. The water is heated. If Bence-Jones proteins are present, at least one tube becomes turbid between 40°C and 60°C, and at temperatures above 65°C, the turbidity disappears (proteins other than the Bence-Jones protein do not become turbid at temperatures up to 65°C). If other proteins are present, the mixture will become significantly more turbid at the boiling point, and the solution is then filtered and cooled. If turbidity then results, the solution is Bence-Jones protein positive.

Results

The Bence-Jones protein was detected at least once in nine of the 64 clients (six females, three males). The three males, however, were positive only once through the entire course, and one (Client 9) of the males was excluded because a definite diagnosis could not be confirmed. Common symptoms exhibited by all but one Bence-Jones protein-positive client (Client 9) included obvious anxiety and disturbances of consciousness that were either transient or lasted several weeks. All of the patients were diagnosed with 'atypishe psychose' (schizoaffective disorder). The Bence-Jones protein was confirmed only at the time when symptoms were worsening and disappeared with improvement. In addition, particularly among five of the six female clients, clear feelings of "Weltuntergangserlebnis" (delusions of negation) were observed midcourse.

In other clinical tests, immunoglobulins (IgG, IgA, IgM, and IgE) were measured and found in five clients. In one of the clients, the levels increased when the symptoms were exacerbated and then abated with improvement. No common features were found in the EEG examinations, but abnormal findings present: the appearance of gentle waves in four of the six clients. Some EEG examinations presented spiked wave patterns.

Discussion and Conclusion

A quantitative testing of the Bence-Jones protein was performed on clients suffering from a schizoaffective disorder. Nine clients were Bence-Jones protein-positive.

Heretofore, it was thought that the Bence-Jones protein was observed only in clients suffering from malignant myeloma. In this study, it was demonstrated that brain phenomena affect not only immune responses but also malignant neoplasms. These phenomena suggest the possibility that schizoaffective disorder displays abnormal changes of malignant neoplasms.

From these observations, we can conclude that brain phenomena affect not only immune responses but also malignant neoplasms.

In this study, for the first time, the hypothesis that there is a relationship among brain phenomena, immune responses, and malignant neoplasms was studied, but the details of this study require further discussion because the details of the relationship between Bence-Jones proteins and malignant myelomas are not clear.

Note: At the time I wrote this article, the editors and publisher did not permit me to publish a discussion, only the results.

References:
Amkraut, A., Solomon, G.F., et al.: Immunoglobulins and Improvement in Acute Schizophrenic Reactions. Arch. Gen. Psychiatry, 28: 623, 1973.

Edelman, G. M., and Gally, J. A.: The Nature of Bence-Jones proteins. J. Exp. Med., 116:207, 1962.

Hazama, H., Kawahara, R., et al.: Immunoglobulins in Schizophrenia Patients. Jap. J. Clin. Psychiatr., 7:475, 1978 (in Japanese).

Hisatome, M. and Miura, Y., Eds.: The Biochemistry of Tumors. Asakura Shoten, Tokyo, 1968 (in Japanese).

Pulkkinen, E.: Immunoglobulins, Psychopathology and Prognosis in Schizophrenia. Acta Psychiatr. Scand., 56:173, 1977.

Stevenson, G. T.: Detection in Normal Urine of Resembling Bence-Jones Protein. J. Clin. Invest., 39:1129, 1960.

Takatsuki, K., and Osserman, E. F.: Fed. Proc., 22:327, 1963: J. Immunol., 92:100, 1964.

Jozuka, H.: Psychoneuroimmunopathology. Maruzen Nagoya, Japan, 2000.

Jozuka, H.: Introduction to Psychoneuroimmunopathology and Clinical Practice. Bibliobooks, 2004.

The Significance of this Study

According to Medard Boss, Hisao Nakai and Bin Kimura, who are prominent psychopathologists in psychosomatic medicine, the phenomenon described in this study could be considered an important advancement in psychosomatic medicine based on psychopathology.

Moreover, this scientific breakthrough may explain the relationship between brain function and malignant neoplasm, including other terminal diseases. This study also laid a foundation for further study on the relationship between immunology and psychopathology.

I wish to explain why and how immunology, neurology and psychopathology have been successfully combined. This method has been practiced for more than thirty years now.

At the time of this study, it was a medical assumption throughout the world that there was no relationship between immune responses and brain phenomena, including brain functions. Furthermore, it was (and is) thought that immune responses and immune functions exist and operate with no relationship to the brain, even if there is evidence to the contrary. Fortunately, when cytokines were found in the brain of a subject for the first time several years ago, studies about relationships between immune responses and brain phenomena appeared in the literature, one after another.

However, I believe that brain phenomena and functions differ deeply from mind and spirit in a human being. Therefore, I wish to include in continuing studies the relationship between the immune response, including all guardian systems, and mind and spirit, which we will call "psychoneuroimmunopathology (PNIP)" in the human being.

The study of psychoneuroimmunopathology began with the study of the relationship between immune responses and psychopathological phenomena. Detailed functions and roles of the Bence-Jones protein are still being clarified in immunology, as far I know. Furthermore, etiological findings of multiple myelomas showing the Bence-Jones protein are available.

I consider the relationship between immune systems and the mind and spirit, including brain functions, to be phenomenologically an existential system.

Primary Research on Psychoneuroimmunopathology

In the early stages, only primitive research was conducted, as described below:

Significantly high IgM levels were found in women with bipolar disorders during manic states.

Significantly high IgE RIST levels were present in people with schizoaffective disorders, particularly during disturbances of consciousness.

Significantly high IgE (RIST and RAST) levels and NK cell activity, and low CD4 and CD8 levels, were found in people with panic disorders before treatment compared to control subjects.

Details are described in the following articles.

1) "Bipolar Disorder Showing High IgM Levels in Manic Stage"
Jozuka, H: Psychiatria et Neurologia Japanica, 1980
Introduction

Although many studies about schizophrenia and immune responses have been performed, no studies of other psychiatric disorders have been conducted for many years. Furthermore, the relationship between endocrino-immunological responses and psychiatric disorders has never been studied.

The IgM values in peripheral blood samples were measured in bipolar disorders to determine the relationship between endocrine responses and psychiatric changes and between immune responses and psychiatric changes. It is well known that IgM levels change along with hormonal changes such as menstruation and pregnancy. Consequently, if IgM levels fluctuate in clients with psychiatric disorders, it would be reasonable to assume that there is a correlation between psychic phenomena, endocrine responses and immune responses.

Subjects and Methods

Serum IgM in the peripheral blood was measured in 32 of the 170 clients who received a consultation in our department of psychiatry in the six months between February 1 and July 31, 1980. IgM was measured four times every month. The 32 clients were suffering from bipolar disorder. No immunological studies into bipolar disorder have been conducted, as far as the authors know, although a number of endocrinological studies have been conducted with bipolar disorders.

The purpose of this study was to investigate the relationship between endocrinological and immunological changes. In particular, IgM levels were measured and compared between female and male clients because females are thought to be more sensitive to hormonal changes.

Results

Thirteen female clients showed high IgM levels at manic stages only, whereas 12 males showed continuously high IgM levels.

Significantly high IgM levels were observed among the 25 clients diagnosed with bipolar disorder compared to the control group.

IgM levels paralleled the menstrual cycle in female patients as follows: high levels of IgM were present approximately 14 days before menstruation began, with IgM levels gradually decreasing as the onset of menstruation approached.

During menstruation, the clients suffered from depressive moods. IgM levels increased, along with mood changes, following menstruation.

No remarkable relationship between changes of IgM levels and mood changes were observed in the male clients.

Discussion and Conclusion

This study represented the first research into the relationships between mood changes, endocrinological changes and immunological changes. Points for discussion arose as follows:

The mood changes accompanying the menstrual cycle are thought to be natural because hormonal fluctuations naturally cause mood changes in females.

The concept of a relationship between changes in IgM levels and mood changes is new. Heretofore, high IgM levels have been associated with inflammation, such as those occurring in autoimmune diseases and other simple inflammations associated with bacterial infections.

Although the manic stage of a bipolar disorder is never an inflammatory state, high levels of IgM were observed in clients only during the manic stage.

Manic moods were clearly related to the menstrual cycle, which relates to hormonal variations.

It was suspected that the mood changes in the female clients suffering from bipolar disorder were related to hormonal variations.

The variations in IgM levels as an immune response were accompanied by mood changes in the females with bipolar disorders.

The changes in IgM levels as an immune response were accompanied by hormonal changes in the females with bipolar disorders.

Although high levels of IgM were observed in the males with bipolar disorder, the high IgM levels were not accompanied by mood changes among the males.

These observations lead us to conclude that there is a close relationship between mood change as a brain function and hormonal phenomena and variations of IgM levels as an immune response. However, it was unclear whether bipolar disorder in males is linked to hormonal change.

These studies show that the brain, hormones, and immune responses are clearly interrelated.

At the time the research was conducted, no comparative studies were available in any area. Today, many similar studies have been performed throughout the world, but I have not compared the results of this study with the results of other similar studies.

Consequently, because the discussions mentioned above were held in conjunction with the actual performance of the study, they are not particularly extensive. However, some discussion continues in light of newer studies, as listed below.

References:

Cruse, M. and Lewis, R. E.: Atlas of Immunology. Springer CRC Press, LLC, New York, U.S.A. 1999.

Jozuka, H.: Psychoneuroimmunopathology. Maruzen Nagoya Japan, 2000.

Maes, M., et al.: Acute phase proteins in schizophrenia, mania and severe depression: modulation by psychotropic drugs. Psychiatry Res. 1997, 66:1-11.

Balatia, C., Iscrulescu C., Sarbulescu, A: Serum immunoglobulin levels in schizoaffective disorders (manic and depressive). Rom J Neurol Psychiatry. 1992, 30:63-7.

Tudorache, B. et al.: Serum immunoglobulin (A, G, M) levels in primary bipolar affective disorders. Rom J Neurol Psychiatry. 1991, 29:35-51.

Bock, E., Weeke, B., Rafaelsen, O. J.: Serum proteins in acutely psychotic patients. J Psychiatr Res. 1971, 9:1-9/

2) "Serum IgE in Schizoaffective Disorder"—*Jozuka, H.: J. Nagoya City Univ. 1982*

Introduction

In 1966, IgE was found in a multiple myeloma and identified as one of the myeloma proteins by Ishizaka, K. et al. Since then, it has been believed that IgE plays a key role in allergic reactions as an immune response. It is also believed that allergic reactions were never controlled by either the brain or psychoneurotic systems.

Among the studies performed in Japan by Kamoshita, I. and Katsura, T. et al. is a report on the suppression of immunoglobulin E (IgE) production under a stress load (1980). To the best of the authors' knowledge, this is the first study to demonstrate the relationship between brain function and IgE. Furthermore, this study was the first to explain that some immune responses are controlled by brain functions (i.e., psychoneurogenetic reactions). The researchers specialized in psychosomatic medicine, particularly in the diseases and physiology of respiratory organs.

Today, it is well known that IgE plays a role in allergic reactions, but IgE was discovered in a malignant myeloma as a myeloma protein. Initially, when IgE was discovered in a malignant myeloma and a multiple myeloma, it was thought that IgE would play some role in the development and advance of neoplasms, but it was later explained that IgE plays a role primarily in allergic reactions.

Since the end of World War II, and only in Japan, there has been a sudden increase in allergic diseases. Prior to the end of World War II, there was no increase in allergic diseases in Japan. It should be noted that no nation in the world, other than Japan, has had to change its traditional staple food. When World War II ended in defeat for the Japanese people, their traditional staple food was no longer available. Consequently, they decided to accept wheat as their new staple food. However, many Japanese people were found to have a wheat-allergic constitution. This fact was explained by the discovery of IgE antigens as the result of a radioallergosorbent test (RAST). The study suggested that other brain phenomena might be caused by changes in IgE levels. Consequently, serum IgE was measured in schizoaffective disorder patients to determine whether it was causing more severe changes in the brain.

Schizoaffective disorder is described as follows:
- In general, this disorder is acute at onset and has a good prognosis but tends to recur.
- The clinical picture is dominated by emotional, consciousness, and psychomotor disorders.
- Polarized symptoms of mania-depression, anxiety-ecstasy, and excitation-stupor are often observed.
- Therefore, studies were conducted on clients suffering from schizoaffective disorders ("Atypishe Psychose") that measured polyclonal IgE levels and specific IgE antigens.

Subjects and Methods

Subjects

The subject group consisted of 158 clients presenting schizoaffective disorder symptoms who visited Toyohashi National Hospital for initial consultations in the four years between February 1, 1980 and January 31, 1984. The authors used the DSM-III in this study.

There were 65 male and 93 female clients varying in age from 20 to 47. Furthermore, after questioning each client or his/her family and after conducting a physical examination at the time of the initial consultation, it was determined that no clients suffered from bronchial asthma, atopic dermatitis, hives or allergic rhinitis. Moreover, after confirming that no medications were being taken, it was determined that none of the clients suffered from allergic diseases.

The control group comprised 20 males and 26 females ages 19 to 39, all of whom had been diagnosed with schizophrenia. A healthy control group of 15 males and 20 females, ages 20 to 48 years, was selected from among the employees at Toyohashi National Hospital.

Methods

After receiving client consent, a 5-ml blood sample was taken, and the RIST (radio-immunosorbent test) was used to determine polyclonal IgE values. The RAST (radioallergosorbent test) was used for specific IgE antigens. There was an extremely large range of specific IgE antigens. For this study, the authors measured house dust (H1, H2) and mites (D1, D2) as year-round allergens; orchard (G) and

Japanese cedar (T) as spring through summer seasonal allergens; and mugwort or wormwood (W) as fall-through-winter seasonal allergens. Thereafter, peripheral blood was sampled in the early morning every alternate week. (When there were obvious changes in the measured values, blood was taken every week for confirmation.)

Concurrent tests on liver and kidney function, hematology, CRP, ASLO, and RA were also conducted.

Results

There were different opinions on the borderline values of IgE (RIST), but the upper limit in the relevant literature is 700 IU/ml, and the authors followed this line. Taking IgE values of 700 IU/ml or above for the highest value of IgE RIST, the results showed 33 clients among the schizoaffective disorder group, two members of the healthy control group, and five in the client control group with RIST values at this level. Using the chi-square test, these values were shown to be significant.

For specific IgE antigen quantification, a semi-quantitative index (maximum index is 4), e.g., expressed by a RAST index, was created using specific IgE serum antigen to white-birch pollen as a control. Determination showed high values of 2.0 or more. In total, 48 clients (30.4 %) from the schizoaffective disorder group, eight from the client control group, and six from among the healthy control group had high values for more than one of the seven types of antigens (called H1, H2, D1, D2, G, W, and T). The values were significant according to the chi-square test. In contrast, no significant difference was observed in the number of clients with RAST values of less than 2.0 among any of the three groups. The relationship between the type of specific IgE antigen and schizoaffective disorder clients with high RAST indexes was as follows: the most common allergens among clients with high values (above 2.0) were the year-round allergens H1, D1, H2 and D2, followed in order by the seasonal allergens T, G, and W. These values were significant according to the chi-square test. (To maintain accuracy, borderline values from 1.0 to 2.0 were excluded).

The relationships between the initial consultation month and the RIST values and the initial consultation month and the RAST values were as follows: the month with highest number of clients with RIST values above 700 IU/ml and the highest number with RAST values above 2.0 was January, followed by September, June and March in this order. However, the distribution of clients with low RIST and RAST values was balanced throughout the year, showing no significant differences.

Clients with both high RIST and RAST values who originally showed clouding of consciousness found that this was alleviated soon after beginning drug therapy. This shows a strong sensitivity to drugs (Haloperidol, Bromperidol, etc.) among clients with high RIST and RAST values. However, lithium carbonate was ineffective in preventing recurrence among those clients with high RIST and RAST values, whereas carbamazepine and sodium valpronic acid were shown to be extremely effective on the whole.

Tests on liver and renal function, hematology, CRP, ASO, and RA were performed to rule out a possible connection of other diseases and RIST and RAST values. At the time of the initial consultation, slight abnormalities were found in these tests for some clients, but within 1 to 2 weeks, all had returned to within the normal range. There were no significant differences in test results among the schizoaffective disorder group, the client control group, and the healthy control group.

In representative cases, high RIST and RAST values were observed only in disturbances of consciousness. High RIST and RAST values gradually decreased and were accompanied by recovery from the schizoaffective disorder.

Discussion: The Relationship Between Schizoaffective Disorders and Allergic Reactions

In the current study on schizoaffective disorders, the authors attempted to measure polyclonal IgE using RIST and specific IgE antibodies using RAST. (Because the same methods and borderline values were used at the time, normal or borderline values differ widely from today's values.) Several points follow for discussion:

The RIST-measured values are polyclonal IgE values, and they are affected by genetic and other factors. Therefore, elevated levels do not necessarily coincide with the presence of an allergic reaction. High IgE blood diseases, along with allergic diseases, include hepatic cirrhosis, acute hepatitis, rheumatoid arthritis, and Kimura's disease. Schizoaffective disorders with elevated serum IgE values must therefore be differentiated from these diseases. In this regard, starting with the initial consultation, the authors performed general blood tests to confirm that there were no singular findings for liver or renal function; furthermore, because there were no CRP, ASO, or RA test findings of note, their contribution for the most part can be ruled out. The fact that such high RIST values were found in a significant majority of schizoaffective disorder clients would therefore suggest a connection with some type of immune abnormality in these clients. For clients not showing high RIST values, the involvement of other immunoglobulins may be assumed, as described elsewhere.

There is reportedly a strong correlation between examinations of specific IgE antibodies using RAST and skin reactions, inhalation inducement tests, P-K response, and other conditions. In other words, there is an extremely high correlation between high RAST values and the existence of allergic reactions. A significant majority of schizoaffective-disorder clients showed RAST values above 2.0, even if only for one type. This strongly suggests the role of some allergic responses in the pathology of schizoaffective disorder clients with high RAST values.

Certain types of allergic diseases such as bronchial asthma, atopic dermatitis, allergic rhinitis, and hives have high RIST and RAST values when they become severe; however, these levels decrease together with the alleviation of symptoms. For the schizophrenic disorders reported here, RIST and RAST values show similar fluctuations. Earlier, the authors reported cases of schizoaffective disorder that became chronic. For these clients, although the RIST values change together with the symptoms, the RAST values showed almost no variation. However, for allergic diseases that have become chronic, RIST and RAST values show almost no change, regardless of changes in symptoms. One cannot, therefore, rule out a connection with allergic reactions in cases of chronic schizoaffective disorders.

Furthermore, Yui has reported on the relationship between symptoms and RIST and RAST values in bronchial asthma clients. According to these reports, the symptoms are at their worst during January, October, June, and March, corresponding to the times when RIST and RAST values increase. From checking and comparing the month of initial consultation with the number of schizoaffective disorder clients having elevated RIST and RAST values, the present investigator found that the greatest numbers of schizoaffective disorder clients with these elevations were recorded in January, followed, in order, by September, June and March. This is strikingly similar to the results of Yui et al. and suggests the existence of similar peaks. In terms of onset, then, one may surmise that there is the same type of seasonality in bronchial asthma as there is with these schizoaffective disorder clients showing high RIST and RAST test results.

For specific IgE antibody titers (i.e., among the schizoaffective disorder group with elevated RAST levels exceeding 2.0), investigation of the type of specific IgE antigen evidencing high RAST levels revealed that year-round antigens such as house dust and mites were most common, whereas seasonal allergens were few. According to Nakanishi et al., in diseases with extreme seasonality, particularly those such as bronchial asthma (including allergic rhinitis), allergens indicating high RAST values are year-round ones such as house dust and mites, followed by seasonal allergens such as Japanese cedar, orchard grass, and mugwort. From this, the authors infer that it is not only the rise and fall of external factors that determines the onset of disease but also the relationships between rising and falling allergens and physical factors for individual clients.

The correlation between RIST and RAST results for schizoaffective-disorder clients is shown as follows: RIST values above 700 IU/ml and RAST values above 2.0 show a significant correspondence. As has previously been described, RIST is hereditary and influences bodily diseases such as hepatic cirrhosis, acute hepatitis, rheumatoid arthritis, and Kimura's disease. Thus, the values do not necessarily reflect the allergic response itself. Therefore, although indirect, RAST values are able to more accurately show the existence of an allergic reaction.

Finally, an important problem remains: the relationship between the brain phenomena of schizoaffective disorder and allergic reactions as immune responses.

On the one hand, schizoaffective disorder is a result of brain phenomena. It has been thought to be caused by fragility of the diencephalons-pituitary axis. Disturbance of consciousness as a basic symptom is a suspected result of the fragility, which, in turn, likely leads to disturbance of consciousness, bipolar disorder-like states and depressive moods and confusion. Some special phenomena are suspected to occur in the brains of schizoaffective disorder sufferers.

On the other hand, high RIST and RAST values were observed only with the existence of symptoms of schizoaffective disorder, as follows: disturbance of consciousness, bipolar disorder-like state, depressive mood and confusion. The results showed that RIST and RAST values corresponded to symptoms of schizoaffective disorder.

This fact led the authors to the conclusion that there is a deep relationship between RIST and RAST values as an immune response and symptoms of schizoaffective disorders as brain phenomena.

Furthermore, Ishizaka, T. et al. first discovered IgE in clients suffering from malignant multiple myeloma. At the time, IgE was considered an immunoglobulin that plays a role in malignant neoplasm, but IgE came to be suspect as having a role in allergic reactions.

From these discussions, the authors concluded that allergic reactions as an immune response can be controlled by the brain. Furthermore, it is suspected that some immune responses may have a significant relationship to deep brain functions.

To the best of the authors' knowledge, such speculations have never been reported until now. The authors will likely be the first researchers to make such speculations.

More detailed explanations are available in "Psychoneuroimmunopathology"[2], which is the first monograph in these areas.

References:
1) Ishizaka, K. & Ishizaka, T.: "Identification of E antibodies as a carrier of reaginic activity". Immunol., 99:1187, 1967.
2) Jozuka, H.: Psychoneuroimmunopathology. Maruzen Nagoya

Japan, 2000.
3) Kimura, B.: The Anthology of Epilepsy. Tokyo Univ. Press.:1980.
4) Johansson, S. G. O., et al.: A new class of immunoglobulin in human serum. Immunol., 14:265, 1968.
5) Bennich, H. et al.: Immunoglobulin E, a new class of human immunoglobulin. Bull. Hlth. Org. 38:151, 1968.
6) Aas, K. & Lundkvist, U.: The radioallergosorbent test with a purified allergen from codfish. Clin. Allergy, 3:255, 1973.
7) Ahlstedt, S. et al.: Specific IgE determination by RAST compared with skin and provocation test in allergy diagnosis with birch pollen, timothy pollen and dog epithelium allergen. Clin. Allergy, 4:131, 1974.
8) Jozuka, H.: "Immunoglobulins in Psychiatry [1]". Psychiatria et Neurologia Japonica 82:737, 1980.
9) Jozuka, H.: "Immunoglobulins in Psychiatry [2]". Psychiatria et Neurologia Japonica 83:597, 1981.
10) Jozuka, H.: "Panic attack and IgE in depressive state". Clin. Psychiat. 25:87, 1983.
11) Kamoshita, I. & Katsura, T.: "IgE levels and psychogenesis in bronchial asthma". Psychosomatic Med. 20:383, 1980.

3) "Panic Disorder and Some Immune Responses"—*Jozuka, H.: J. Psychiatry, 1989*

Introduction

As molecular immunology has developed, the existence of humoral immunity controlled by immunoglobulins and cellular immunity controlled by lymphocytes has become clearer. Humoral immunity is differentiated from B cells and controls the function of creating antibodies with immunoglobulins such as IgG, IgA, IgM, IgD, and IgE. It is commonly said that cellular immunology performs a cytotoxic (killer) function. A landmark development in cellular immunology has occurred. Not only was a new immune cell discovered but new ground has also been broken for elucidating immune junctions. Within the short space of a few years, even clinicians can obtain measured values very readily.

In this connection, the DSM-III was published, and lymphocytes, particularly T lymphocytes, have been actively measured for schizophrenia in Europe and the United States, with a variety of reported results. However, in the beginning, there were many reports of the inability to obtain consistent results because of elementary mistakes such as differences in measured values (depending on the facility). Even after these problems were rectified, the results ranged from an increase in immune function to a decrease. Today, perfectly consistent results remain elusive. This appears to reflect differences that depend on the specific time at which results are obtained over the long term with schizophrenia.

In everyday treatment, the authors encounter a great deal of "panic disorder." The specific symptom of this disorder is a panic attack, and as with atypical psychological phenomena, it is characterized by "attack."

The diagnostic criteria for this disorder are as follows:

At least three panic attacks within a three-week period in circumstances other than during marked physical exertion or in a life-threatening situation. The attacks are precipitated by more than just exposure to a circumscribed phobic stimulus.

Panic attacks are manifested by discrete periods of apprehension or fear, and at least four of the following symptoms appear during

each attack:
- Dyspnea
- Palpitations
- Chest pain or discomfort
- Choking or smothering sensation
- Dizziness, vertigo, or unsteady feelings
- Feeling of unreality
- Paresthesia (tingling in hands or feet)
- Hot and cold flashes
- Sweating
- Fainting
- Trembling or shaking
- Fear of dying, going crazy, or doing something uncontrolled during an attack

Not the result of a physical disorder or another mental disorder, such as severe depression, somatization disorder, or schizophrenia.

The disorder is not associated with agoraphobia.

According to these criteria, IgE was first measured, followed by the measurement of T lymphocytes (and subsets, including natural killer cell activity).

Subject Group 1 (who were measured for IgE) and Methods
Subjects

The subjects were 90 clients whose main symptom was panic attacks who made their first visit to the Toyohashi National Hospital Psychiatric Outpatient Clinic during a two-year period from November 1, 1979 to October 31, 1981. Their ages ranged from 19 to 53 years. The authors did not differentiate between sexes because it is believed that there are no gender-specific differences in IgE. The DSM-III was used for diagnosis. Tests were performed on a control group comprised 33 healthy staff members at Toyohashi National Hospital.

Methods

For polyclonal IgE, RIST (radioimmunosorbent test) was performed using the "IgE kit 1"; the specific IgE antibody assay was scored (4.0) with specific IgE antibody serum (References A, B, C, D) on white-birch pollen as a control using RAST (radioallergosorbent test). (For H1 and H2, house dust extract from Pharmacia Co. was used.)

Results

In 11 clients, high values greater than 700 IU/ml were found for IgE RIST, showing significant difference from the control group. Furthermore, a significant correlation was found between high IgE levels and panic disorder. All patients experienced either a panic attack and/or an acute disturbance of consciousness as a major symptom. Common points were not always found in the electroencephalographic findings, but slow bursts were noticed in many cases. Clients given IgE RIST tests exhibited abnormally high values of 2-4 for allergy specific antigens such as house dust (H1 and H2) and dust mites (D and F).

Of course, many clients have never experienced allergic diseases such as bronchial asthma, atopic dermatitis, and allergic rhinitis.

Discussion

Panic disorder and schizoaffective disorder are included in the "Krise" (crisis) category identified by Plugge, mentioned above as schizoaffective disorders. Similar immunological concepts that apply to discussions about clients suffering from panic disorders may also apply to those suffering from schizoaffective disorder.

Among clients for whom it was possible to run an IgE RIST and RAST, high values were found when the panic attack was severe, and these values decreased as the symptoms alleviated. This variation in IgE RIST and IgE RAST values matched variations in clients who had certain types of allergies, such as atopic dermatitis, hives, or bronchial asthma. When the attacks occurred frequently for clients with certain types of bronchial asthma and when swelling, redness, or itchiness appeared for clients suffering from dermatitis, the IgE RIST and IgE RAST values increased, and when the symptoms alleviated, the values also decreased. The appearance of sudden redness and swelling, which accompany unbearable itchiness for dermatitis sufferers, and sudden coughing attacks, which accompany fear of death for bronchial asthmatics, have been reported.

In other words, the aforementioned atopic dermatitis and bronchial asthma attacks are non-psychological, i.e., they require physical means to resolve the psychological condition specified as anxiety. These conditions (the swelling and redness that accompany sudden itchiness for dermatitis and the fear of sudden death for bronchial asthma attacks) that the authors call a panic attack can also be termed what Kimura, B. calls the "intra festum" (in a festival or during festival) mechanism, from the German psychopathological specification we call "paroxysmal."

When "festum" is called a festival, it usually has a before, during and after stage. Although "festum" has been defined as the ideation of existential philosophy, it has a very similar meaning to festival in English philosophy. "Ante festum" is an attitude similar to "before the festival," which indicates anxiety about what will happen in the future. "Post festum" is an attitude similar to "after the festival," which indicates some depressive mood in an irretrievable state. "Intra festum" has an attitude of attack and crisis, such as during the middle of a festival.

These discussions led the authors to the conclusion that IgE is the immunological substance explaining the severity of crisis, paroxysm, and attack.

Subjects and Future Methods
From December 1, 1997 to November 30, 1998, CD3, CD4+, CD8+, and natural killer cell activity was measured in 85 clients suffering from panic disorder between 09:00 and 10:00 A.M. at their initial consultation. A 60-person normal control group was also tested. It was determined that these clients and the control group had never suffered from bacterial and viral infections, inflammatory diseases, neoplasm, autoimmune diseases, or hepatitis.

Peripheral blood was collected between 09:00 and 10:00 A.M. Within 24 hours, CD3, CD4 and CD8 levels were measured by the radioimmunoassay use of monoclonal antibodies. Natural killer cell activity was measured with a chromium-51 (^{51}Cr) release test using $Na_2{}^{51}CrO_4$.

Results

In clients suffering from panic disorder, the authors measured mature T lymphocytes (CD3+) and their subsets, helper/inducer T lymphocytes (CD4+), suppressor/cytotoxic T lymphocytes (CD8+), and natural killer cell activity (NK cell activity).

Table 1 shows the results of measuring these immune cells for panic disorder.

Panic Disorders (n=85)	Controls (n=60)	
CD3+ (%)	63.58±8.99	74.56±14.35*
CD4+ (%)	34.16±7.56	46.85±9.98*
CD8+ (%)	36.48±8.02*	28.15±7.17
NK cell activity (%)	5.21±2.51*	3.59±1.94
t-test:*p<0.01		

Table 1: T cell Line and NK Cell Activity Test Results For

Description of Table 1: T cell, subsets, and natural killer cell activity were measured in clients suffering from panic disorder when panic attacks occurred frequently. The results showed significantly low levels of CD3+ and CD4+ and significantly high levels of CD8+ and natural killer cell activity.

In panic disorders, when panic attacks (one of the main symptoms) occurred frequently, specific immune responses were found:

CD3+ showed significantly lower levels.
CD4+ showed significantly lower levels.
CD8+ showed significantly higher levels.
Natural killer cell activity showed significant higher levels.

Discussion and Conclusion

A discussion of the T-cell results should be separate from that of the natural killer cell activity because the immune functions for each differ.

On the one hand, T cells are derived from hematopoietic precursors that migrate to the thymus where they undergo differentiation and continue to completion in the various lymphoid tissues throughout the body or during their circulation to and from these sites. The T cells are primarily involved in the control of the immune responses by providing specific cells capable of helping or suppressing these responses. They also have a number of other functions related to cell-mediated immune phenomena.

The T-lymphocyte subpopulation is a subset of T cells that have a specific function and express a specific cluster of differentiation (CD) markers or other antigens on their surface. Examples include the $CD4^+$ helper T-lymphocyte subset and the $CD8^+$ suppressor/cytotoxic T-lymphocyte subset.

On the other hand, natural killer cells attack and destroy certain virus-infected cells. They constitute an important part of the natural immune system, do not require prior contact with an antigen, and are not MHC restricted by the major complex histocompatibility system that expresses cytotoxicity against various nucleated cells, killer (K) cells, or antibody-dependent cell-mediated cytotoxicity (ADCC) cells that induce lysis through the antibody action. Immunologic memory is not involved because previous contact with an antigen is not necessary for NK cell activity. In addition to their ability to kill selected tumor cells and some virus-infected cells, they also participate in antibody-dependent cell-mediated cytotoxicity (ADCC) by anchoring antibodies to the cell surface through an Fc -receptor.

As mentioned above, T cells and their subpopulations differ immunologically from NK cell activity.

Panic attacks in panic disorders are included in 'Krise' (crisis) in the pathological attitude. Furthermore, it is suspected that panic attacks are psychopathologically categorized into "intra festoon," instead of before the attack in "ante festoon."

When panic attacks occur frequently, brain phenomena are in crisis and intra festum. This situation belongs to the resistance stage according to the "Stress Theory" by Selye, H.

In such a state, immune responses become established as the human being's defense. As a result, the immune response becomes a significant factor in natural killer cell activity because NK cell activity does not require prior contact with an antigen.

These reactions are often considered psychosomatic. The authors define such phenomena as a psycho-neuro-immuno-pathological human defense mechanism.

References:
1) Cruse, J. M. & Lewis, R.E.: Atlas of Immunology. CRC Press LLC USA, 1999.
2) Selye, H.: The Stress of Life. McGroaw-Hill Paperbacks, 1978
3) Ceuppens, J. L., et al.: The presence of Ia antigen on human peripheral blood T cell and T-cell subsets. Cell Immunol. 64:277-292, 1981.
4) Hoffman, R. A., et al.: Simple and rapid measurement of human blood. Proc. Natl. Acad. Sci. USA 77:4914-4917, 1980.
5) Reinherz, E. L. et al.: Separation of functional subsets of human T cells by monoclonal antibody. Proc. Natl. Acad. Sci. USA. 76:4061-4065, 1979.
6) Kronfol, Z., House, J. D.: Depression, cortisol, and immune function. Lancet 8384:1026-1027, 1984.
7) Baker, G. H., et al.: Stress, cortisol, and lymphocyte subpopulations. Lancet 8376, 574, 1984.

"Psychopathological problems were suspected through these studies, which is why the connection between immune responses and psychopathological problems was studied in the first place."

Experimental Studies

The following experimental studies were conducted:

- The relationship between Rorschach tests and immune responses
- Immune responses to severe stress
- Changes in immune responses to related stressors
- Immune responses on Type A behavior patterns.

Experimental Study #1: Variations in IgE Levels Before and After Rorschach Tests
Introduction
It was believed that an allergic reaction will lead a person who has a congenital allergic predisposition to develop allergic diseases such as bronchial asthma, atopic dermatitis and rhinitis and that only IgE, which is one of the myeloma proteins, plays a role in the allergic reaction. Furthermore, allergic reactions are believed to be peripheral reactions. As a result, the concept that allergic reactions relate to brain function has been ignored throughout the world.

However, only one race in the world has had to suddenly change the staple food in its diet. As expected with such a change, allergic rhinitis and other allergic diseases have dramatically increased in the Japanese, who were forced to change their staple food after they lost a war.

Since this sudden change in diet occurred, research about allergology as a peripheral reaction has increased, but to this day, the relationship between brain functions and allergic reactions has been ignored.

Recently, the psychosomatic approach has become the most common treatment. Before such phenomena became apparent, psychosomatic experiments were conducted on ordinary people.

The Rorschach test is a well-known personality test and is actually the most easily understood test of personality. However, to achieve a true understanding of the client's personality, the client must be willing to open up his or her heart. In other words, "open heartedness" will affect catharsis. Usually, under ordinary circumstances, people are very reluctant to open their hearts. Although people often wish to open their heart, they are not always able to do so because of their need to protect and guard themselves against other people.

People do open their hearts during Rorschach tests. The Rorschach test might be a unique opportunity to disclose their suppressed and hidden inner world.

Subjects and Methods
Subjects
The subjects were six ordinary people on the hospital staff who had never taken the Rorschach test and had no prior knowledge of the test.

Methods
The elements of this experiment were as follows:

Measurements of IgE RIST (radioimmunosorbent test) values and serum cortisol were performed 10 minutes before the Rorschach test was administered.

The Rorschach test was performed. Because the length of time differs for each person, time was not limited.

Measurements of IgE RIST values, including serum cortisol, were performed immediately after the Rorschach test.

The "Baum" test (tree drawing test) was performed before and after the Rorschach test.
Results
The results of this study were as follows (see Figures 1 and 2):

IgE RIST values were significantly decreased after the Rorschach test compared to before (*p<0.01).

Serum cortisol showed a significant decrease after the Rorschach test compared to before (*p<0.01).

Although the "Baum test" (tree drawing test) reflected a natural style before the Rorschach test, the "Baum test" appeared as a grape tree after the Rorschach test.

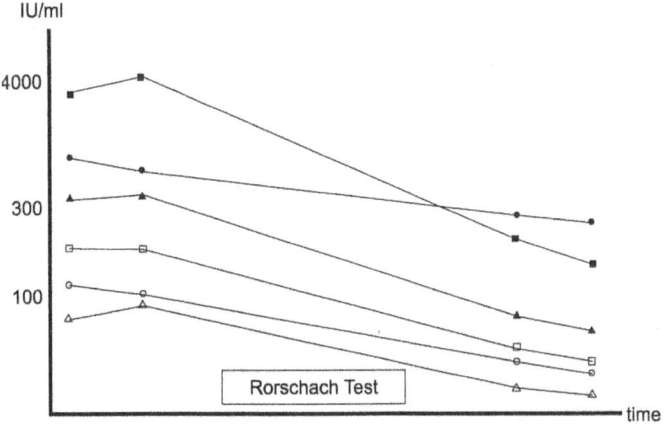

Figure 1: Serum IgE levels before and after Rorschach test as catharsis (n=6)

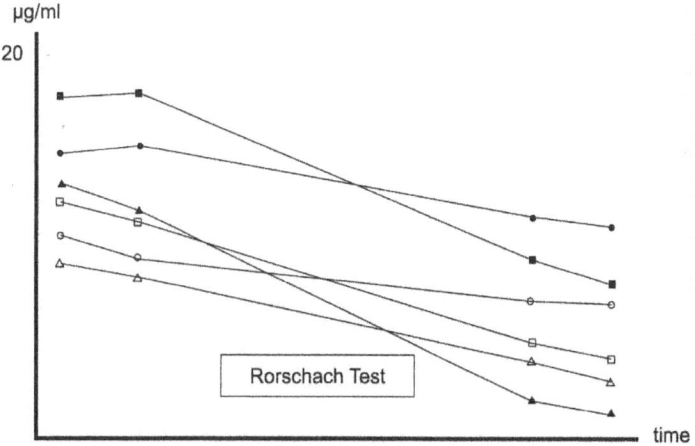

Figure 2: Serum cortisol levels before and after Rorschach test as catharsis (n=6)

Discussion and Conclusion

In this study, IgE RIST values and serum cortisol decreased because of the Rorschach test, which allowed a catharsis of the client's inner world and resultant relaxation. The catharsis of the inner world indicates that the clients were able to open their hearts. When a person's suppressed inner-world is expressed, even if it occurred unconsciously, he or she will become deeply relaxed. The Rorschach test plays the role of relaxation therapy.

Relaxation induced by the Rorschach tests decreased the IgE values relative to the client's level of relaxation. When people become non-protective and non-suppressive, their IgE values decrease. From these findings, we understand that not only somatic but also psychological relaxation can reduce IgE values. When IgE values are decreased, allergic reactions will not occur as easily.

This leads us to the conclusion that catharsis is one of the methods that should be used to treat allergic diseases such as bronchial asthma, atopic dermatitis, and allergic rhinitis.

Until now, it was believed that increased levels of pollens aggravated allergic diseases. Consequently, only protection from pollens was used as a preventive measure against allergic diseases. As a result of this study, the main treatment to reduce IgE values will involve various means of psychological catharsis including relaxation and play therapy for children.

These observations led us to the conclusion that it is important to treat allergic diseases through the use of psychoneuroimmunological therapies.

References:

Tamkin, A. S.: Rorschach Card Rejection and Its Relationships to Defensiveness, Intelligence, and Sex. Psychol. Rep. 44:1003-1006, 1979.

Yanovski, A. & Fogel, M. L.: Visual Imagery Reactivity: Relationships to Rorschach Responses, Diagnostic Classification and Therapeutic Potential. Psychol. Rep. 45:1003-1010, 1979.

Frank, G.: On the validity of hypotheses derived from the

Rorschach: V. The relationship between from level and ego strength. Perceptual and Motor Skills 48:375-384, 1979.

Ellenberger, H. F.: The Discovery of the Unconscious. Basic Books, A subsidiary of perscus Books, LLC, 1981.

Exner, J.E. Jr., Wylie, J.: Some Rorschach data concerning suicide. J Pers Assess. 1977, 41:339-48.

"Unconscious catharsis occurred through the use of Rorschach tests."
"The experiment investigated the suspected relationship between immune responses and psychopathological phenomena, including personality."

Experimental Study 2: Responses to Acute and Intolerable Treadmill Stress

Introduction

It is well known that the various responses that are observed depend on each stressor, as discussed in the "Stress Theory" by H. Selye.

Furthermore, it is also well known that responses to a sudden stress differ from responses to chronic stress. In a sudden stress situation, humans show acute resistance reactions, but in continuous, chronic stress, humans show other defensive reactions. However, it has never been clarified which type of stress causes which type of response, even at an endocrino-immunological level.

In such situations, the authors considered it important to clarify all responses in the stages outlined in the "Stress Theory."

This experiment was conducted to study the psycho-neuro-endocrino-immunological responses of ordinary persons in a sudden and intolerable stress situation, in accordance with the "Stress Theory."

The treadmill is used to check for hidden heart failure by exerting stress on the client's heart. It is considered one of the most useful examinations used by heart specialists. However, this method has also been called a torture machine because the stress that it generates becomes intolerable. In this experiment, the treadmill was used to exert acute short-term stress, and some endocrino-immunological responses were evaluated. Some psycho-neuro-endocrino-immunological discussion will occur along with a description of the experiment.

*This experiment was conducted as part of a company health promotion plan, which was devised to promote employee health in the company after the death rate had become too high and had spiraled out of control.

Subjects and Methods

This experiment was conducted at the NTT Nagoya Health Administration Center in July 1998.

Subjects:

Twelve individuals who had no history of heart failure or inflammatory disease participated in the experiment. The participants also had no complaints about their state of mind and body, were in good health, and had been working every day for more than three months. These 12 people participated on a voluntary basis. They were all males aged 26 to 32. They willingly cooperated with this study. The participants were general employees and not specialists in their fields and worked for Nippon Telephone and Telegram Co. Ltd.

Methods:
Natural killer cell activity and cortisol were measured 30 minutes before, immediately before, immediately after, 30 minutes after and 60 minutes after using the treadmill. The Bruce method was used on the treadmill. Natural killer cell activity was measured using the Separated method, which involves ^{51}Cr. Both parameters were measured within 24 hours after taking a blood sample.

When the first measurement of cortisol was made, general chemical tests were also performed on the blood to confirm that there were no abnormal findings in the subjects' peripheral blood.

Results
The results of the experiment are illustrated for natural killer cell activity in **Figure 1** and serum cortisol in **Figure 2**.

Natural killer cell activity was significantly elevated immediately after use of the treadmill, and natural killer cell activity gradually decreased in relation to elapsed time (t-test: $p<0.01$).

Cortisol significantly increased immediately after use of the treadmill and decreased in relation to elapsed time (t-test: $p<0.01$).

Discussion and Conclusion
Natural killer cell activity and serum cortisol showed significant elevation after the acute and sudden stress of the treadmill test. These responses are very similar to the resistance stage reaction to stress as defined by H. Selye. Natural killer cell activity and serum cortisol might provide the explanation for higher levels at the resistance stage of stress.

During short-term and acute stress, natural killer cell activity and serum cortisol can show severe elevations.

These phenomena led to the conclusion that acute stress elevates natural killer cell activity and serum cortisol values.

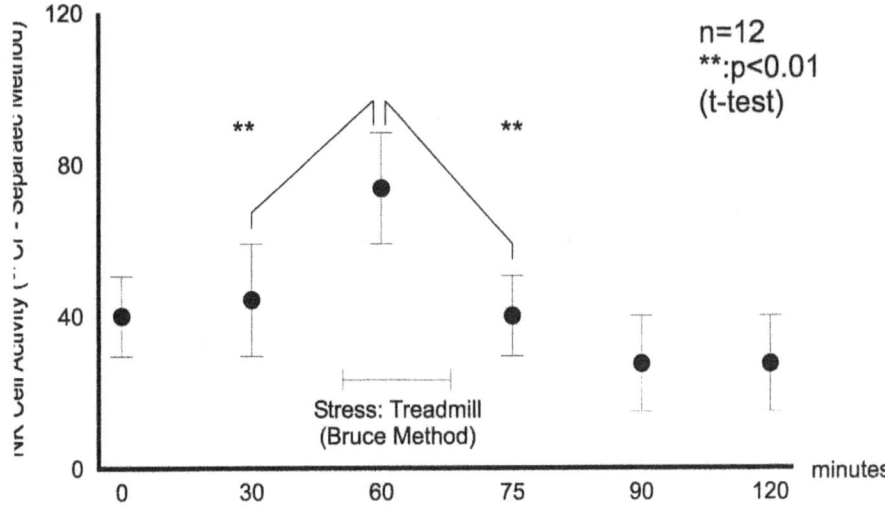

Figure 1: Variation of natural killer cell activity in a short-period stress (treadmill)

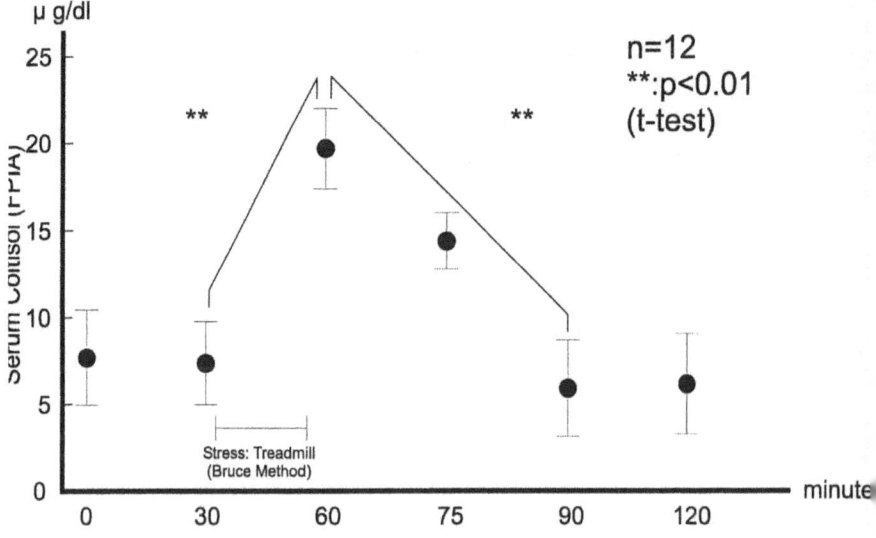

Figure 2: Variation of serum cortisol levels in a short-period stress (treadmill)

Natural killer cells play a role in providing initial protection in the face of sudden and acute stress because MHC is not restricted by the major histocompatibility complex (MHC) antigens.

Any sudden stress and/or antigens in a human being can promote natural killer cell activity.

Observation of the natural killer cell activity and cortisol responses show that they can both be considered actions of the first defense systems.

Endocrino-immune responses are increased in response to new stress with which the person has never had previous contact.

Under short-term stress, people show severe reactions, but the reactions gradually fall into the range of an ordinary state of stress.

Human beings show immediate and acute reactions to stress but recover almost immediately and return to an ordinary state. It is suspected that such reactions occur only under short-term and sudden stress.

This study shows that human reactions depend on the type of stress that is exerted and its duration.

References:

1) Cruse, J. M., and Lewis, R. E.: Atlas of Immunology. Springer CRC Press LLC USA, 2000.
2) Selye, H.: The Stress of Life. McGraw-Hill Paperbacks, 1978.
3) Messina, G., et al.: A psychoncological study of lymphocyte subpopulations in relation to pleasure-related neurobiochemistry and sexual and spiritual profile to Rorschach's test in early or advanced cancer patients. J Biol Regul Homeost Agent. 2003, 17:322-6.
4) Messina, G., et al.: Efficacy of IL-2 immunotherapy in metastatic renal cell carcinoma in relation to the psychic profile as evaluated using the Rorschach test. Anticancer Res. 2007, 27:2985-8.

"This occurrence explains the psychosomatic defense mechanism against a sudden and harsh change in human homeostasis. The results showed the psychosomatic nature of immune responses."

Experimental Study #3: Responses to Sudden Short-Term Stress and to Duplicate Stresses

Introduction

The relationship between human beings and stress has been studied, but it is well known that human responses differ depending on the person's state of mind and body and on the stressor, i.e., in what type of situation the human was subjected to which type of stressor.

Studies by previous researchers were conducted using ordinary persons who had willingly volunteered to participate in the studies.

For more than 20 years, one male volunteer had been donating a blood sample once a month except when there were special circumstances or accidental stress. In this instance, specific reactions were observed for 2 years (from 1989 to 1991) of the 20-year period. The specific reactions are defined as immune responses and endocrinological responses.

The development of immunological parameters has been steadily increasing. In this situation, variations in natural killer cell activity and serum cortisol are illustrated in the following chart.

One Volunteer's History (Figure)

Case: Forty-five-year-old male; head manager of the largest company in the country.

The volunteer is a 45-year-old male. He has been the head manager of his department for approximately five years. He willingly participated in this study because he has been interested in the research performed by the authors.

His work, ideas, and abilities were highly valued by the president of the company. One day he was supposed to go with his immediate supervisor to meet with the president to discuss a new project. His boss permitted the volunteer, in his capacity as Department head manager, to accompany him to the meeting, but would not allow him to say one word (a common phenomenon in Japan). Following the discussion, his boss not only began to ignore him but also stopped giving him work.

In addition, his boss spent a day and a night inventing a mistake that he (the volunteer) had supposedly made at work. Although he had actually made no mistake in the work, his boss suddenly gave him notice to resign. He was surprised, and repeatedly exclaimed, "Why? What happened?" He came running into the author's office exclaiming loudly, "Check my body, and check my blood!"

His natural killer cell activity and serum cortisol were measured immediately. Both values were extremely elevated compared to his usual values (**1st stress in Figure**). The high values gradually decreased after several months.

He was again given notice when he was immersed in his most important work. He was surprised and exclaimed, "Why, again?" He visited the author and said loudly, "Check my blood!"

His natural killer cell activity and serum cortisol were measured immediately. Both parameters were severely elevated again (**2nd stress in Figure**). Over several months, the parameters gradually decreased to his usual levels.

From then on, his boss frequently called him into his office and gave him notice to resign. This occurred repeatedly.

He frequently visited the author for counseling and to donate his blood samples. He looked very tired and complained that he was too tired to work. This feeling of tiredness, which began when his boss started giving him frequent notices to resign, gradually worsened.

His natural killer cell activity and serum cortisol were measured in all of these situations. The results showed responses opposite to his healthy reactions. Immediately following a stressful encounter with his boss, his natural killer cell activity and serum cortisol values showed significantly lower levels than the volunteer's usual values under normal conditions. Furthermore, his usual levels of both parameters began to show lower and lower values than those shown after the first measurements (**3rd and 4th stresses in Figure**).

Fortunately, he was invited to be a vice-president in the major company. He decided to accept the invitation immediately. From then on, his natural killer cell activity and serum cortisol parameters gradually increased to levels similar to the first measurement (**at 2nd year in Figure**).

Three years after receiving the invitation to become vice-president, he became the president of the company. Although the president's duties are likely to be very stressful, he was so healthy that both parameters showed values similar to those of the first measurement. He said, "I am leading a very comfortable life every day. No one will ever try to threaten my position. This is my greatest peace."

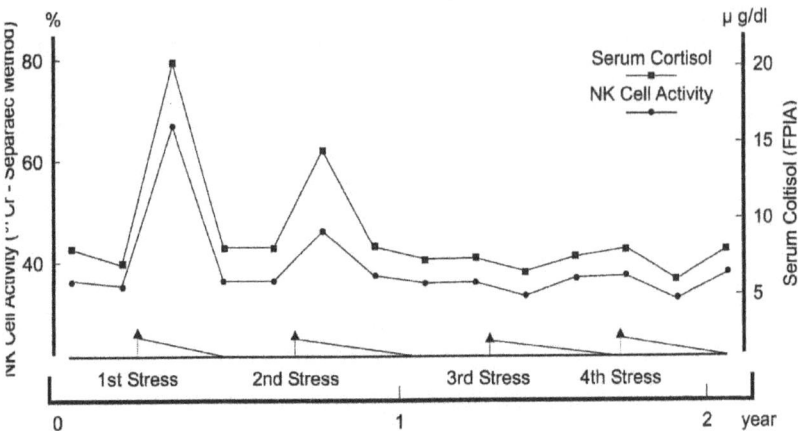

Figure: Variation of natural killer cell activity and serum cortisol in long-term stress of two years in a 45-year-old volunteer

Description of the Figure

Variations in natural killer cell activity and serum cortisol levels are shown in this graph. Severe elevations of the natural killer cell activity and serum cortisol levels were observed at the first stress. At the second stress, both parameters showed a slightly lower elevation. At the third and fourth stresses, both parameters showed lower than ordinary levels, when the volunteer was in an exhausted state. After fully recovering his health, both parameters gradually became elevated.

Discussion and Conclusion

Measurements of natural killer cell activity and serum cortisol were performed frequently on the male volunteer under various circumstances. The responses of natural killer cell activity and serum cortisol have been outlined as follows:

Under ordinary circumstances, his natural killer cell activity and serum cortisol values were nearly identical.

His natural killer cell activity and serum cortisol values elevated at the first sudden stress.

His elevated natural killer cell activity and serum cortisol values gradually decreased after the stress return to their usual levels.

His natural killer cell activity and serum cortisol values suddenly elevated again when he was exposed to the same stress a second time.

His higher natural killer cell activity and serum cortisol values gradually decreased over the course of several months.

When he encountered frequent stress, he gradually became very tired. While he was suffering from this extreme tiredness, his usual natural killer cell activity and serum cortisol levels decreased until they were lower than the first measurement.

When he became very tired, although he was exposed to the same stress, his natural killer cell activity and serum cortisol showed further reduction.

After embarking on a new career move that gave him a new life, his psychosomatic situation improved more and more. Simultaneously, the values of both parameters became very similar to the original levels taken at the first measurement.

From the abovementioned responses, it can be observed that even similar stresses or the repetition of the same stress generates different reactions in a person. When a person is in a healthy and active state, he will display sudden defensive and protective responses. As a result, natural killer cell activity and serum cortisol might elevate because of the sudden stress. However, when a person becomes exhausted because of the frequent and continuous stress, his defense mechanism might also become exhausted. As a result, the natural killer cell activity and serum cortisol might show a reduction because of frequent stress.

A healthy and active state appears to be a protective state, and an exhausted state is similar to the state of exhaustion as defined by Selye.

When measurements were performed at the two-year period, the relationship between immune responses and corticosteroids was commonly suspected, but it was not commonly accepted that interleukin-2 (IL-2) promotes natural killer cell activity. Of course, corticosteroid and interleukins have never been shown to be correlated previously.

On one hand, Selye identified elevation of corticosteroids as a result of stress. At the time, it was believed that elevated corticosteroids promoted elevated immune responses. On the other hand, it was thought that corticosteroids do not always promote immune responses; in some situations, corticosteroids elevate immune responses, and in other situations they suppress immune responses. In their studies, the authors reached the conclusion about these different ideas that corticosteroids promote interleukin-2, which promotes natural killer cell activity and reduces the T-cell line (T cell and subsets).

These observations led the authors to the conclusion that when a person is in a healthy and active state, natural killer cell activity and cortisol will elevate as primary protective responses, but in an exhausted state, the protective mechanism cannot react in the body and mind. Instead, in this situation, the T-cell line might be expected to elevate only to the level of bare necessity for defense.

This has led to the common conclusion that immune and endocrinological responses might be aroused depending on the state of mind and body of the human being. Because such situations in a human being are not always stable, the immune and endocrine response will be unstable in exactly the same manner.

References

Jozuka, H.: Psychoneuroimmunopathology. Maruzen, Nagoya, Japan, 2000.
Selye, H.: The Stress of Life. MacGroaw-Hill Paperbacks, 1978
Cruse, J. M. & Lewis, R. E.: Atlas of Immunology. CRC Press LLC USA, 1999.

"The high elevation of NK cell activity due to sudden short-term stress was apparent at the first incident, and as the same stress was repeated, the responses were gradually reduced."

Experimental Study #4: Immune Responses in Type A Behavior Patterns

Introduction

Immune responses have been thought to differ depending on personality and/or behavior patterns. For example, the Type C personality is commonly known to be more prone to certain types of cancers than the non-Type C personality. The schizoid personality might be defensive immunologically. It is well known that "Typus Melancholicus" (the melancholic type of personality), as defined by Tellenbach, will become depressed more easily. This personality might easily reduce immune responses because superficial protection is the extent of its defenses. The protection mechanism of this personality might be fragile.

Furthermore, natural killer cell activity, IL-2, serum cortisol and DHEA (dehydroepiandrosterone) were significantly decreased in severe depression compared to the control group.

A psycho-neuro-endocrino-immunological study was performed on subjects with Type A behavior patterns to consider the type of situations common to persons of a Type A behavior pattern. There will be some accompanying discussions relating to this study.

Subjects and Methods

Subjects:

The subjects were 79 male volunteers who work for a major company. The Jenkins Activity Survey (JAS) was used to type-classify their behavior patterns. The Type A group included 36 persons aged 32.93 ± 4.80 years, and the Type B group included 43 persons aged 34.72 ± 8.37 years. There was no significant difference between the Type A and Type B behavior pattern groups.

Methods:

The methods were as follows: the immunological parameters CD4, CD8 (T cell subsets) and natural killer cell activity and the endocrinological parameters serum cortisol and thyroxin were measured at 9:00 am on March 10, 1989.

The measurement of CD4 and CD8 was performed using monoclonal antibodies. Natural killer cell activity was measured using the ^{51}Cr-Separated method.

In addition to these measurements, CRP, RA, ASLO, liver function, renal function, pancreas function, white blood cell and red blood cell tests results were all found to be within normal limits. Furthermore, the subjects had not suffered from any inflammatory diseases during the previous 4 weeks.

Results

The results of this study were as follows:

In CD4, the Type A group (25.51±7.4 %) showed significantly (t-test: *p<0.01) higher values than the Type B group (16.31±7.25 %).

In CD8, the Type A group (5.44±2.54 %) showed significantly (t-test: *p<0.01) lower values than the Type B group (11.16±4.27 %).

In natural killer cell activity, the Type A group (22.06±6.38 %) showed significantly (t-test: *p<0.01) higher values than the Type B group (15.33±9.28 %).

In serum cortisol, the Type A group (14.87±6.54 g/ml) showed significantly (t-test: *p<0.01) higher values than the Type B group (10.67±5.28 g/ml).

In thyroxin (T4), the Type A group (10.53±1.26 g) showed significantly (t-test: *p<0.01) higher values than the Type B group (8.07±1.18 g/ml).

Discussion and Conclusion

On the one hand, T-cell lines are suppressed in Type A personalities compared to the activated natural killer cell activity that functions as an immune response. On the other hand, thyroid function and adrenal function were activated in Type A persons.

The Type A behavior pattern is characterized as more severe, hostile, unyielding, and impetuous, with workaholic tendencies, compared to Type B. It is suspected that persons with Type A behavior, who have such tendencies, are always in the resistant stage as defined in the Stress Theory by Selye, H. As a result, immune and endocrinological responses might display higher levels than in Type B individuals. Furthermore, persons with Type A behavior patterns have psycho-neuro-endocrino-immunologically similar defense mechanisms against sudden and acute stress. They exist, as such, in a treadmill situation as previously described.

In the short term, Type A people will never consciously reach a resistant state. The overall results make this abundantly clear.

Immunologically, Type A people are defined as being on the offensive, as explained by elevated values of the natural killer cell activity. Endocrinologically, serum cortisol plays a protective role. The Type A behavior pattern consumes more energy than Type B. High levels of thyroxine in Type A persons verify this fact.

In the short-term, the Type A behavior pattern is useful in the workplace, but in the long-term, the energy levels of Type A individuals will not endure. As a result, Type A people will not suffer from any diseases because of immune and endocrinological responses in the short-term, but in the long-term, the strong Type A individual will become weakened because of long-term fatigue.

Crises tend to occur suddenly to Type A people. Such a crisis generally occurs when the Type A person suddenly relaxes and/or becomes fatigued.

Furthermore, because the Type A subjects showed lower levels of CD8, it is suspected that Type A individuals will be weak at preventing bacterial infections because the T-cell line requires prior contact with antigens to develop protection against them. Consequently, Type A individuals will need to rest to fight against bacterial antigens and viral antigens. Type A individuals always have offensive abilities against viral antigens but do not have protective abilities against bacterial antigens.

From these observations, Type A individuals require relaxation and rest to prevent diseases that do not require prior contact.

Therefore, people who exhibit severe Type A behavior patterns must draw close to a Type B person to enjoy a psycho-neuro-immunologically healthy life. They must change not only their behavior pattern but also their basic lifestyle.

References:

Ader, R., Felten, D., Cohen, N.: Psychoneuroimmunology, 2nd Ed., New York, Academic Press, 1992.

Eysenck, H. J.: Anxiety, learned helplessness, and cancer: A causal theory. J. Anxiety Disorders, 1:87-104, 1987.

Tellenbach, H.: Melancholie, Springer, Berlin, 1961.

Jozuka, H., et al.: Comparison of Immunological and Endocrinological Markers Associated with Severe Depression. J. Int. Med. Res. 31:36-41, 2003.

Jenkins, C. D., Zyzanski, S. J. & Rosenman, R. H.: Jenkins Activity Survey, Psychological Co-Op, New York, 3-31, 1979.

Friedman, M. & Rosenman, R. H.: Association of specific overt behavior pattern with blood and cardiovascular findings. JAMA 169:1286, 1959.

Hayano, J., Jozuka, H., Fujinami, T., et al.: Type A behavior pattern in Japanese employees: cross cultural comparison of major factors in Jenkins Activity Survey (JAS). J. Behav.Med. 12(3):219, 1989

"From a psychopathological and immunological point of view, these results mean that Type A persons are always in a lifestyle of struggle."

Experiments Related to Treatments

Experiment Related to Treatment #1: Psychoneuroendocrinoimmunopathological responses of SSRI
Introduction
It has usually been reported that life-supporting mechanisms such as psychological, endocrinological, and immunological mechanisms are reduced during severe depression.

Reduced immune responses and adrenal corticosteroids show lower values in subjects suffering from severe depression than in those of the control group.

On one hand, such a report might give the impression that the treatment of depression using SSRIs will immediately be effective in elevating these responses. On the other hand, SSRIs might elevate the functioning of defense mechanisms including endocrinological functions in ordinary persons, whereas other antidepressants might elevate endocrinological and immunological responses only in depressed subjects who have already displayed lower levels.

From these points of view, measurements of immune and endocrinological responses in normal persons were conducted to understand variations brought about by SSRIs.

Subjects and Methods
Subjects:
Fifty-six employees of a major company volunteered to participate in this study. They had never suffered from depression and had no inflammatory diseases, liver function diseases, renal diseases, or other chronic diseases during the previous month. This was determined by psychological tests and peripheral blood tests as shown below. Additionally, they willingly cooperated with these studies after giving their informed consent. They showed SDS scores (Self-rating Depression Scale by Zung) of less than 30 points.

The volunteers were general employees and did not hold special positions in their office.

Methods:
The natural killer cell activity (NKCA) and interleukin-2 (IL-2) productivity were measured as immune responses, and serum cortisol, dehydroepiandrosterone (DHEA) and dehydroepiandrosterone-sulfate (DHEA-S) in the peripheral blood were measured as endocrinological responses. These measurements were taken before, one month after, and two months after taking the SSRI Fluvoxamine at a dosage of 50 mg/2/day. In addition to the measurements mentioned above, CRP, ASLO, and RA were always found to be within normal limits.

The subjects promised to abstain from alcohol for these two-month periods.

Results
The results are illustrated in the accompanying Figures.

Natural killer cell activity showed significant elevation after taking the SSRI compared to the results before taking it (t-test: *$p<0.01$, Figure 13).

The interleukin-2 productivity index showed significant elevation after taking the SSRI compared to the results before taking it (t-test: *$p<0.01$, Figure 14).

Serum cortisol showed significant elevation after taking the SSRI compared to the results before taking it (t-test: *$p<0.01$, Figure 15).

Dehydroepiandrosterone showed significant elevation after taking the SSRI compared to the results before taking it (t-test: *$p<0.01$, Figure 16).

Dehydroepiandrosterone showed no significant change in the results before and after taking the SSRI.

During these two months, no remarkable changes were observed in the results of the other tests mentioned above. Furthermore, none of the diseases mentioned above were observed during these two months.

Discussion

Because of developments in immunology, immunological parameters have increased. Therefore, discussions must be considered in greater detail than before.

The results of the tests showed that fluvoxamine as an SSRI was clearly effective in elevating the capacity for the endocrino-immunological response in ordinary persons. However, it might be claimed that we do not have precise data when reductions of endocrino-immunological parameters were caused by depression and that the use of SSRIs to recover from depression reduced parameters that were elevated as a result.

Although the parameters were measured in ordinary subjects, they were altered by the SSRIs. Therefore, SSRIs have the ability to change parameters. Discussion must be established from this starting point, i.e., the discussion should focus on the effects of SSRIs.

Natural killer cell activity, which is promoted by interleukin-2, was elevated by SSRIs in ordinary normal people and is accompanied by elevation of the interleukin-2 productivity index. These phenomena show that SSRIs not only have the ability to elevate the reduced immune responses of depression but also have the definite ability to elevate immune responses.

On the one hand, some researchers report that cortisol does not always elevate immune responses but suppresses them at times. As a result, it cannot always be concluded that elevated cortisol caused the increase in immune responses.

On the other hand, dehydroepiandrosterone has always displayed a repair and recovery role. It is possible that immune responses were elevated because of elevated dehydroepiandrosterone due to the SSRIs.

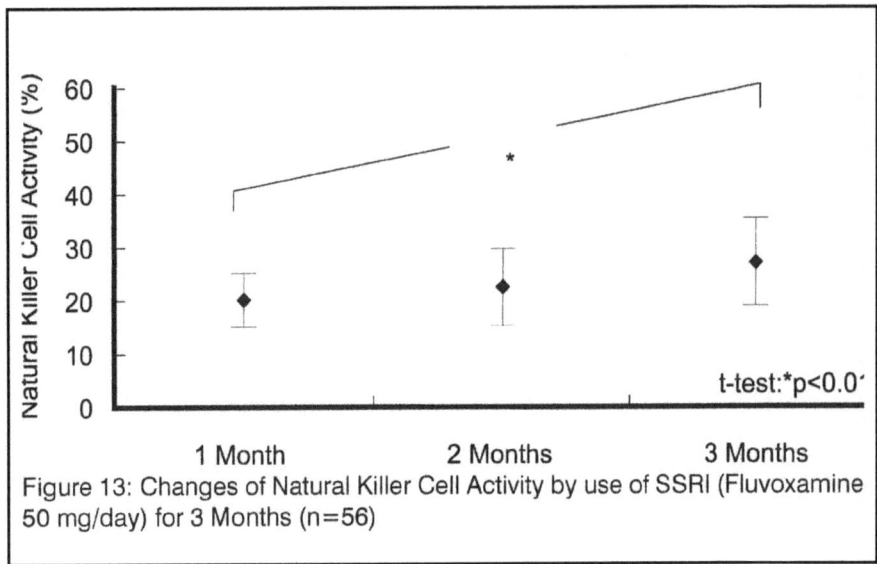

Figure 13: Changes of Natural Killer Cell Activity by use of SSRI (Fluvoxamine 50 mg/day) for 3 Months (n=56)

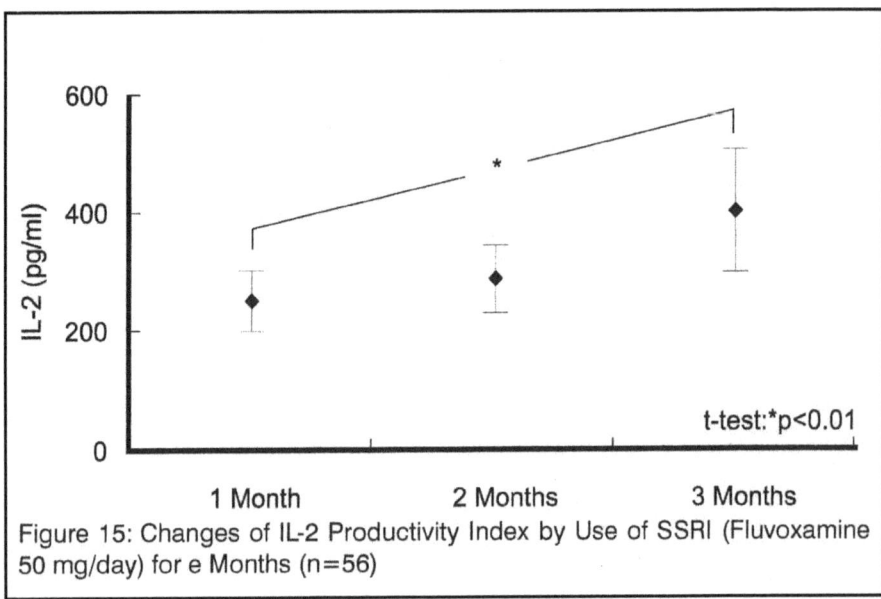

Figure 15: Changes of IL-2 Productivity Index by Use of SSRI (Fluvoxamine 50 mg/day) for e Months (n=56)

The graphs above have been reproduced from the original study.

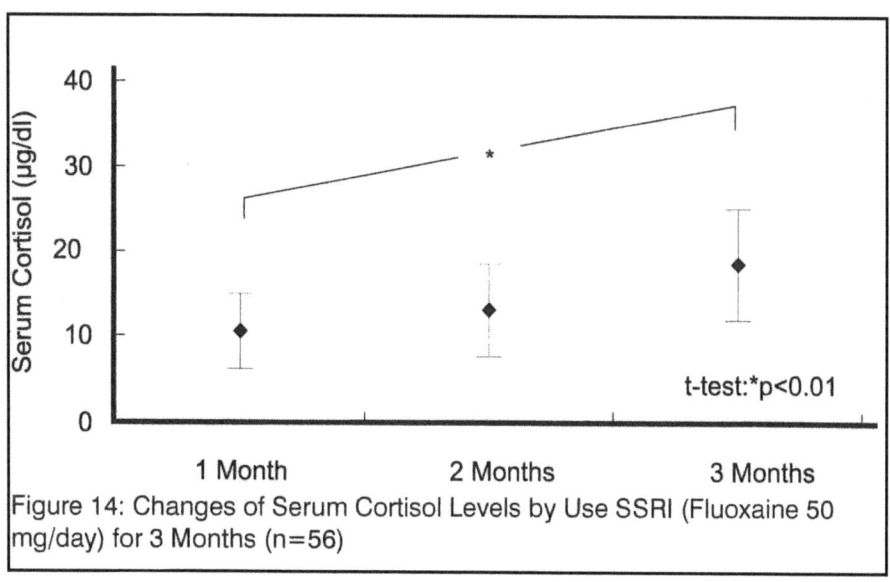

Figure 14: Changes of Serum Cortisol Levels by Use SSRI (Fluoxaine 50 mg/day) for 3 Months (n=56)

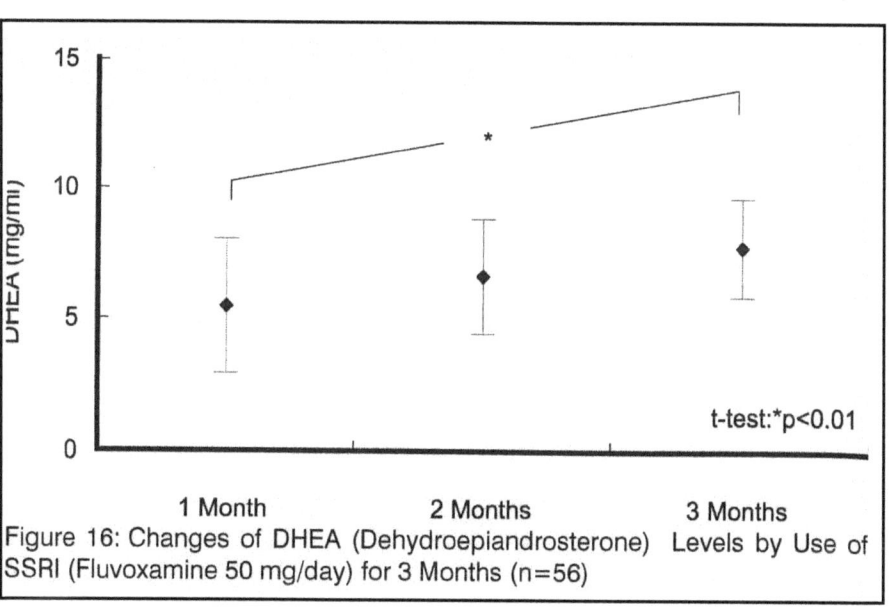

Figure 16: Changes of DHEA (Dehydroepiandrosterone) Levels by Use of SSRI (Fluvoxamine 50 mg/day) for 3 Months (n=56)

The graphs above have been reproduced from the original study.

Furthermore, the SSRIs might lead directly to the elevation of immune responses by affecting the brain. As a result, interleukin-2 is elevated, and the natural killer cell activity is enhanced by the SSRIs. Natural killer cells attack and destroy certain virus-infected cells. They constitute an important part of the natural immune system, do not require prior contact with antigens, and are not MHC antigens. Natural killer cells are lymphoid cells of the natural immune system that express cytotoxicity against various nucleated cells, including tumor cells and virus-infected cells.

These observations led the authors to conclude that SSRIs may have tumor destroying abilities, including the repair and recovery functions of dehydroepiandrosterone. However, the relationship between immune responses and endocrinological responses remains unclear. It would be valid to conclude that natural killer cell activity, including interleukin-2 productivity, might be influenced by dehydroepiandrosterone due to SSRIs.

Another opinion notes that dehydroepiandrosterone has the ability to elevate immune responses, particularly in defense lines. Furthermore, it plays a role in tumor apoptosis.

Conclusion

These observations led us to conclude that SSRIs have the ability not only to elevate natural killer cell activity and interleukin-2 but also to manage dehydroepiandrosterone. Therefore, SSRIs have the ability to prevent and destroy neoplasms with dehydroepiandrosterone.

References

Nishikaze, O. & Furuya, E.: Stress and Clinical Examinations. Clin. Pathol. 42:321-330, 1994.

Nishikaze, O. & Furuya, E.: Stress and Anticortisol Hormone. J. Industrial Medical School, 20:273-295, 1998.

Frank, M. G., Hendricks, S. E., Johnson, D. R., Wisseler, J. L. & Burke, W. J.: Antidepressants augment natural killer cell activity: in vivo and in vitro. Neuropsychology 39(1):18-24, 1999.

4) Loria, R. M., Padgett, D. A. & Huynh, P. N.: Regulation of

the immune response by dehydroepiandrosterone and its metabolites. J. Endocrinol. 150: S209-S220, 1996.
5) Cruse, J. M. & Lewis, R. F.: Atlas of Immunology. CRC Press, LLC USA, 1999.
6) Loria, R. M.: Immune up-regulation and tumor apotosis by androstene steroids. Steroid 67:953-966, 2002.
7) Evans, D. L., et al.: Selective Serotonin Reuptake Inhibitor and Substance P Antagonist Enhancement of Natural Killer Cell Innate Immunity in Human Immunodeficiency Virus/Acquired Immunodeficiency Syndrome. Biol Psychiatry. 2000.

"Those results showed that SSRIs might be not only antidepressants but also anticancer and antiviral agents. However, it was not proven that SSRIs directly stimulate immune mechanisms or recovery from depression, but immune abilities were elevated subsequent to taking SSRIs."

Experiment Related to Treatment #2: Psychoneuroendocrinoimmunopathological Responses of Laughing Training"

Introduction

At the 12th International College of Psychosomatic Medicine convention in 1993, psychosomatic responses, particularly endocrine-immunological responses because of laughing, were discussed in one of the symposiums.

Since this symposium, research into psychosomatic responses to laughter training and therapy has been conducted worldwide.

Today, the conclusion is that laughing both creates and maintains good health. It is therefore important to laugh for good health. Following this symposium, many methods for inducing laughter were applied in different medical areas. It has been said, "Laughing leads to a happy life;" thus, laughter therapy has come under discussion as a specific method. Laughing appears to be similar to catharsis, which can be explained concretely. In other words, laughing appears to be an emotional release. If so, many psychobiological changes in human beings will be discovered during laughter training. In human beings, being open-hearted creates health.

Furthermore, it was reported that laughter therapy elevated natural killer cell activity. As a result, laughter therapy was thought to be effective in treating some forms of cancers.

From these standpoints, endocrino-immunological studies were conducted on healthy persons to determine changes because of laughter.

Subjects and Methods

Subjects:

Fifty-six healthy volunteers (28 males and 28 females) employed by the previously mentioned major company ranging in ages from 25 to 43 years old were included in this study. The subjects were suffering not only from inflammatory diseases but also from other significant diseases. Their SDS (Self-rating Depression Scale) gave them a reading of less than 30 points.

Methods:

As an immunological study, natural killer cell activity and interleukin-

2 productivity indices were measured before and after the laughter training.

As an endocrinological study, serum cortisol and dehydroepiandrosterone levels were measured before and after the laughter training.

As a determination of the state of their health, white blood cells, red blood cells, CRP, ASLO, RA, liver function, renal function, pancreatic function, cholesterol and triglycerides levels were also measured.

The laughter training consisted of a professional comedian performing for approximately one hour.

Results

Natural killer cell activity and interleukin-2 were significantly elevated compared to values before the laughter training: **Figures 1 and 2** (t-test: *$p<0.01$).

Serum cortisol and dehydroepiandrosterone were significantly elevated compared to values before the laughter training: **Figures 3 and 4** (t-test: *$p<0.01$).

No significant abnormality was observed in white blood cells, red blood cells, CRP, ASLO, RA, liver, renal or pancreas function, or cholesterol and triglyceride levels.

During the laughter training, the volunteers laughed continuously.

Discussion and Conclusions

Laughter is a positive human behavior as far as this experiment is concerned. Human beings laugh only when their hearts are open. Human beings never laugh in stressful situations. Laughing is exactly the eustress (pleasant or curative stress) that humans need.

In this study, the subjects were relaxed and enjoyed the performance. The endocrino-immunological responses as noted below were observed in these experiments. Additionally, although it is commonly thought that laughter is not unusual for human beings, the laughter training showed unusual responses in peripheral blood tests.

In this study, natural killer cell activity was significantly elevated during laughter. Many researchers worldwide have reported that

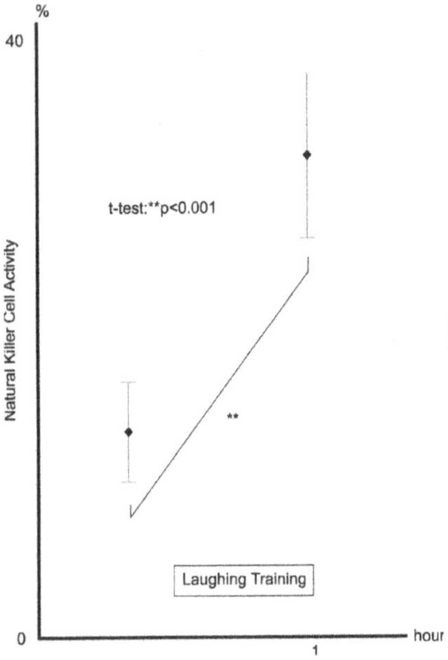

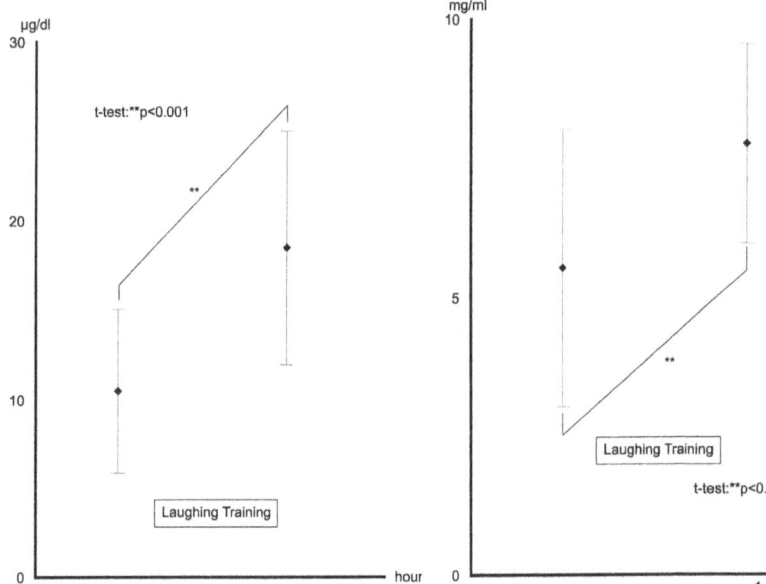

Figure 17: Changes of natural killer cell activity during a laughter training for one hour (n=54)

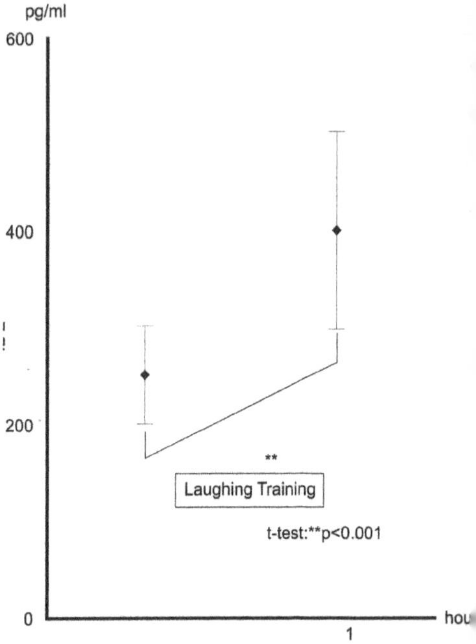

Figure 18: Change of IL-2 productivity levels during a laughter training for one hour (n=54)

Figure 19: Changes of serum cortisol levels during a laughter training for one hour (n=54)

Figure 20: Changes of DHEA (dehydroeplandrosterone) levels during a laughter training for one hour (n=54)

laughter therapy elevates natural killer cell activity. Corresponding with this result, serum cortisol and dehydroepiandrosterone also showed higher values. On the one hand, serum cortisol does not always activate immune responses. At times, cortisol suppresses immune responses. On the other hand, the higher dehydroepiandrosterone levels always activate immune repair and recovery factor responses.

Furthermore, higher values of interleukin-2 were observed during the laughter training that also influenced the susceptible cytokine circuit.

These observations led the authors to conclude that laughter training elevates natural killer cell activity, the cytokine circuit, and the adrenal cortex functions. These phenomena are closely related to one another.

Natural killer cells, which are enhanced by interleukin-2, destroy virus-infected cells and neoplasm cells.

This results in speculation that there is a brain-adrenal cortex-immune systems axis.

Laughter therapy might be effective for the prevention and treatment of cancers, if one considers the role of natural killer cell activity, interleukin-2, and dehydroepiandrosterone.

Laughter training will be one of the forms of health-generating training to prevent neoplasms in human beings because of the elevated levels of natural killer cell activity, interleukin-2, and dehydroepiandrosterone, which has a repair and recovery role.

However, when the natural killer cell activity is elevated, the T cell line shows a reduction. The T cell line is responsible for the destruction of bacteria-infected cells. As a result, a problem will remain with bacterial infections. Clients suffering from neoplasms never have such problems.

References:
Basse, P. H., Whiteside, T. L., Chambers W., et al.: Therapeutic activity of NK cells against tumors. Int. Rev. Immunol. (Switzerland), 20 (3-4):439-501, 2001.
Bennett, M. P., Zeller, J. M., Rosenberg, L., et al.: The effect of mirthful laughter on stress and natural killer cell activity. The

Altern Health Med. (United States), 9 (2):38-45, 2003.

Cruse, J. M. & Lewis, R. E.(eds.): Atlas of Immunology. New York: CRC Press: 23-58, 185-206, 1998.

Cousins, N.: Anatomy of an Illness. New York NY; W. W. Norton 1979.

Berk, L. : Eustress of mirthful laughter modifies natural killer cell activity. Clinical Research 37:1989.

Walsh, J. : Laughter and Health. New York NY: Appleton, 1928.

7) Christie W., Moore C.: The impact of humor on patients with cancer. Clin J Oncol Nurs. 211, 2005

"It was proven that laughter therapy increases immune abilities and DHEA levels."

Experiment related to Treatment #3: Psychoneuroendocrinoimmunopathological Responses to Autogenic Training

Introduction

Although a great deal of research exploring the relationship between immune responses and relaxation is available, the results are often inconsistent. Many reports hold that relaxation increases the immune response whereas other reports conclude that relaxation suppresses the immune response. Other researchers found that relaxation elevates some immune responses and suppresses others.

Such varying results and phenomena have been reported because the conditions under which the measurements were obtained were not determined in advance. For example, in a subject suffering from exhaustion, natural killer-cell activity might show elevated levels, whereas in an aggressive and healthy person, natural killer-cell activity might show lower levels as a result of relaxation, in accordance with the Stress Theory.

This study was conducted to determine which types of immune responses are suppressed by relaxation in subjects in various conditions. The relationship between natural killer cell activity and relaxation therapy was confirmed in the first round of this study.

Subjects and Methods

Subjects:

The subjects were 12 able-bodied male medical representatives (age: 29.6±6.8) in a major pharmaceutical company. They were all very active and healthy Type A personalities and therefore had not had any diseases during the previous five years. They willingly participated in this study.

Methods:

For one year, the 12 volunteers underwent autogenic training once a week in a room at the author's clinic. This training is a type of relaxation therapy that is commonly practiced in psychosomatic medicine.

From the beginning of the study, autogenic training was performed three times a day during this period. Each history sheet confirmed this.

The levels of natural killer cell activity as an immune response and serum cortisol as an endocrinological response were measured at 9:00 am before the autogenic training and before the autogenic training in the first week of each month.

In the first week of every month, a blood sample was taken to determine whether any of the 12 volunteers had suffered from any inflammatory diseases during the week. Furthermore, ALT, AST, LDH, ALP, -GTP, creatinine clearance, BUN, total cholesterol, triglyceride, white blood cells, red blood cells, Hb, Ht, and platelets were also measured every time a blood sample was taken.

Before the first measurement was taken for this study, both the natural killer cell activity and serum cortisol were measured when diffuse slow -waves patterns were observed in the EEG. At the time, both parameters showed the lowest levels measured throughout the entire experiment.

Results
The results of this study were as follows:

Autogenic training was performed throughout nearly the entire period of the study.

The variation in natural killer cell activity is illustrated in **Figure 1**. The natural killer cell activity gradually decreased over the year. A significant reduction was observed between the first and the last values (t-test: *$p<0.01$).

The variation in serum cortisol is illustrated in **Figure 2**. The serum cortisol values gradually decreased over the year. A significant reduction was observed between the first and the last values (t-test: *$p<0.01$).

The results of further blood samples were completely within normal limits.

Discussion and Conclusions
It is usually believed relaxation, including autogenic training, elevates natural killer cell activity and reduces serum cortisol. However, although serum cortisol decreased, natural killer cell activity also decreased in this study. These results differ from many of the previous reports.

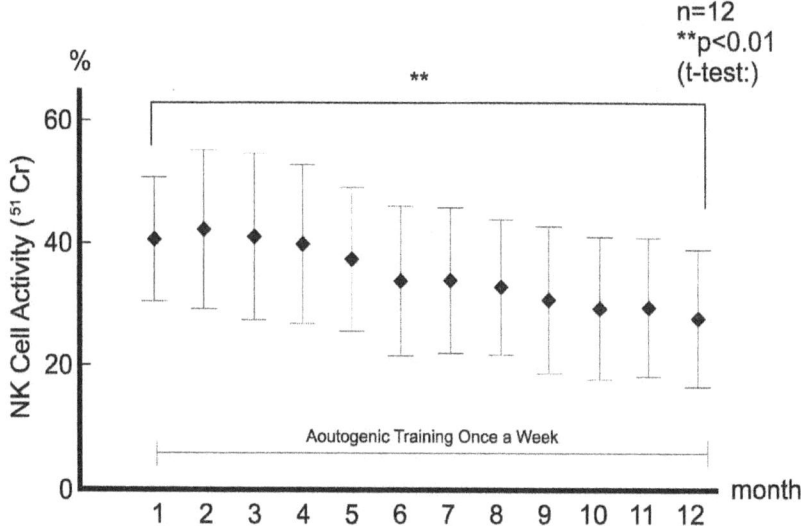

Figure 1: Variation of natural killer cell activity in ordinary persons performing autogeneic training for one year

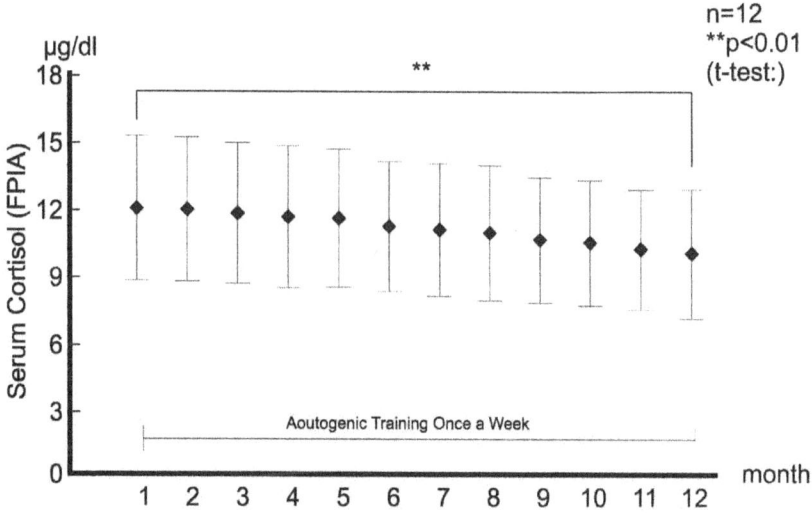

Figure 2: Variation of serum cortisol levels performed autogeneic training in ordiinary persons for one year

On the one hand, it was commonly believed that natural killer cell activity is elevated when serum cortisol increases, but in fact, the opposite pattern actually occurred.

On the other hand, elevations of both natural killer cell activity and serum cortisol were observed in the initial reaction to a stressor, in accordance with Selye's Stress Theory, which was described previously.

Furthermore, at the Stress Theory "resistance stage," it is natural that both parameters become elevated.

If these problems had been clarified when this study was performed, different and unexpected data would have been dealt with more easily.

When the personalities and situations of the subjects were clearly defined, the unexpected responses that were observed correlated with those facts.

When those responses were analyzed, it became evident that if the personality type is clarified first and the subjects' life situation is defined, then the resultant responses are significant.

It is likely that all of the 12 volunteers were active and under constant stress because they worked in the sales department, which is a competitive environment. They were likely excited, stressed, active, etc. Such situations can be defined as the "resistance stage." As a result, personality types and situations are accurately clarified and defined in similar and/or the same patterns.

Based on the above observations, it is natural that both parameters showed higher levels because their customary lifestyle is more stressful than relaxed. It is also natural that both parameters gradually decreased as a result of the autogenic training for relaxation.

Because the 12 volunteers were in an unusual situation, both parameters were elevated before performing autogenic training. Why did both parameters decrease as a result of the autogenic training? The answer is easy and clear: neither parameter was reduced; they both simply returned to their normal ranges.

From this point of view, it is speculated that although the 12 volunteers were considered ordinary individuals, their psychosomatic mechanisms were likely abnormal and psycho-pathologically unhealthy. Because the 12 volunteers showed higher natural killer cell activity and serum cortisol because of their unhealthy psychosomatic mechanism, i.e., they were hyperactive and over-defensive, they entered the "exhausted stage" very easily. If they remain in this situation, they might suffer not only from cancers but also from other viral infections because of the reductions in natural killer cell activity and serum cortisol.

This study clarifies that an "ordinary person" is not always a healthy person. At times an "ordinary person" can also be unhealthy. There will always be opportunities for additional experiments.

"Finally, if all of the volunteers were Type A behavior personalities, this study shows that autogenic training would help develop healthy habits and prevent most diseases."

References:

1) Lindberg, D..A.: Integrative review related to meditation, spirituality, and the elderly PMID. Geriatre. Nurse 26, 372, 2005.

2) Elsenbruch, S., et al.: Effects of mind-body therapy on quality of life and neuroendocrine and cellar immune function in patients with ulcerative colitis. Psychother Psychosom. 74, 277, 2005.

3) Christie W., Moore C.: The impact of humor on patients with cancer. Clin J Oncol Nurs.: 211, 2005.

4) Naito, A., et al.: The impact of self-hypnosis and Joherei on lymphocyte subpopulations at exam time: a control study. Brain Res Bull: 241, 2003

5) Gruzelier, J. H.: A review of impact of hypnosis, relaxation, guided imagery and individual differences on aspect of immunity and health. Stress 5: 145, 2002.

Kmiec, Z.: Cooperation of liver cells in health and diseases. Adv Anat Embryol Cell Biol. III-XIII, 2001.

Hosaka, T., et al.: Effects of a structured psychiatric intervention on immune function of cancer patients. Tokai J Exp Clin Med. 25,: 183, 2000.

Naliboff, B. D., et al.: The effects of opiate antagonist naloxone one measure of cellar immunity during a rest and brief psychological stress. Psychosom Res.39, :345, 1995.

Jozuka, H.: Introduction to Psychoneuroimmunopathology and clinical practice. Biblio-books, Israel, 2004.

Experiment Related to Treatment #4: Comparison of Immunological and Endocrinological Markers Associated with Severe Depression

Depressed clients are usually more susceptible to cancers than normal clients. The authors will demonstrate this fact in this immuno-endocrinological investigation performed on subjects suffering from severe depression.

From Jozuka, H. et al.: J. of International Medical Research vol. 31, 2003©

Introduction

The role of the immune system in mental diseases has been shown by Jozuka (1-5), Masek et al. [6] and Webster et al. [7] There is evidence of a bi-directional relationship between the brain and the immune system. [8] The presence of various indicators of immune activation has been demonstrated in depressed patients. (9-11) Depressed patients display an increased number of T cells in an early phase of activation. [12] In addition, severe depression has been shown to be accompanied by decreased serum activity of dipeptidyl peptidase IV, a membrane-bound serine protease that catalyzes the cleavage of various cytokines and neuro-active peptides stimulating T-cell activation and the production of cytokines, such as IL-2. [13] Various direct and indirect indicators of a moderate activation of the inflammatory response system, particularly an increased production of proinflammatory cytokines, [14] have also been reported. Jozuka (2-5) has suggested that the reduced activity of the body's initial defense system, including the innate immune response as represented by NK cell activity, and the increased activity of the body's secondary defense system or cellular immunity represented by T cell activity, are immune characteristics of severe depression.

DHEA is produced in the brain and adrenal cortex and is believed to be involved in cellular repair and recovery. (15-18) Specifically, it is thought to maintain nerve cell function in brain tissue and to promote immune function in peripheral tissue. [16] Low morning DHEA levels may be associated with severe depression, at least in adolescents. [19]

The aim of the present study was to compare NK cell activity and serum cortisol levels as indicators of the body's initial defense system and IL-2 levels as indicators of cellular immunity in patients with severe depression in comparison to controls. Furthermore, endocrine mechanisms, particularly measurements of DHEA and DHEA-S, were evaluated in patients with severe depression in comparison to controls.

Subjects and Methods
Subjects:
The study included 17 patients (9 women and 8 men) who were diagnosed with severe depression according to the DSM-III-R at the Jozuka Mental Clinic from October 1994 to September 1998. The patients were selected based on a first depressive episode. They had received no treatment at the time the first blood samples were obtained, and they were all free of allergic or infectious reactions for at least 2 weeks prior to blood collection. The aim of the study was explained to the patients, and informed consent to participate was obtained from each patient. The patients ranged in age from 23 to 54 years (mean ± SD = 40.3 ± 15.1). The healthy control group consisted of 10 people (6 women and 4 men) of a similar age range from 23 to 51 years (mean ± SD = 39.9 ± 9.8) with no history of mental disorders; this group comprised welfare volunteers and clinic staff. No difference in the weight of the subjects was observed between the two groups.

Methods
Blood was collected between 9:00 and 10:00 A.M. Within 24 hours, NK cell activity was measured by a 51Cr discharge test using Na251CrO4. (20, 21) IL-2 was measured with a commercial ELISA kit by a tube-fixation method using several monoclonal antibodies that identify different epitopes of human IL-2 within the range of 50-1,600 pg/ml. Cortisol, DHEA and DHEA-S levels were determined using radioimmuno-assays. [22]

The Zung Self-rating Depression Scale [23] was used to evaluate the severity of depressive symptoms.

Results

As expected, the patients with severe depression had a higher SDS score than the healthy controls (Table 1); moreover, the NK cell activity was lower and the IL-2 levels were significantly higher in the patients with severe depression than in the healthy controls (Table 1). Cortisol and DHEA levels were significantly lower in the depressed patients than in the controls (Table 1). No significant difference was observed in DHEA-S levels between the patients and controls (Table 1).

Discussion

In the present study, NK cell activity and IL-2 levels were measured as indicators of immune activity, and serum cortisol, DHEA and DHEA-S were measured as indicators of endocrine function.

The reduction of NK cell activity found in patients with severe depression is in agreement with earlier observations. (24-26) The enhancement of IL-2 in depressed patients may be a compensatory response to the reduced NK cell activity. (see 27, 28) As Carson et al. [29] discussed, it would be very dangerous for a living organism not to compensate for this decreased first-line defense (NK cell activity).

However, the fundamental question remains of whether depression causes the immune and endocrinological changes or whether they are the cause of depression. There is some evidence to suggest that treatment with IL-2 and interferon-alpha can induce depressive symptoms and activation of the inflammatory response system. [30] Antidepressants have negative immunoregulatory effects both in vitro and in vivo, which would be consistent with their antidepressant efficacy being, at least in part, related to their immune effects. [14]

Hyperactivity of the hypothalamic-pituitary-adrenal (HPA) axis and increased cortisol levels are well documented in depression. (31, 32) Both Stein et al. [33] and Miller et al. [34] have reported increased serum cortisol levels in patients with severe depression. We have no explanation for the discrepancy between these results and those found in this study. Cortisol levels vary considerably depending on the time of blood collection, the mental state of the person and the period of time after the onset of severe depression. [2] Thus, cortisol levels are likely the least reliable markers of those measured in this study.

DHEA promotes the synthesis of IL-2 and interferon-g and inhibits the suppression of IL-2 and interferon-g synthesis by glucocorticoids (35,36). Nishikaze and Furuya [16] suggest that DHEA, through its antagonism of glucocorticoids, acts as an anti-stress agent that facilitates tissue recovery (37,15,17). In fact, there is evidence to suggest that DHEA acts to cause tumor regression. (35,36). In psychiatry, Goodyer et al. [19] have suggested that low morning DHEA levels may be associated with severe depression, at least in adolescents. In addition, when patients suffering from severe depression were treated with DHEA, improvements were observed in their depressive symptoms [38]. Thus, the decrease in DHEA observed here in depressed patients may be a cause or a consequence of their depression.

DHEA-S exists in large amounts compared to DHEA; thus, it is difficult to observe changes of the order of those observed here in DHEA. DHEA-S levels are thought to change substantially only just before death when they display a large decrease. [15]

As discussed above, it appears reasonable to postulate that there may be a link between the decreases in NK cell activity and DHEA levels and the increase of IL-2 found in patients with severe depression. Again, however, the question of cause or consequence is pertinent. Because depressed mood has been associated with reduced NK cell activity, some investigators have studied the effect of antidepressants on this parameter. Serotonin, which is thought to be implicated in the pathophysiology of affective disorders, enhances NK cell activity in vitro, and lymphocytes possess serotonin transporters and receptors. [39] These authors have evaluated NK cell activity in depressed patients before and after treatment with the selective serotonin reuptake inhibitor (SSRI), fluoxetine, and also the possible direct effects of SSRIs on NK cell activity in vitro with lymphoid cells. The SSRI was found to enhance NK cell activity not only in vivo (in patients, with amelioration of their depressive symptoms compared to healthy controls) but also in vitro. This latter observation suggests a possible direct drug interaction with lymphocytes. Helgason et al. [40] found similar results in vitro with paroxetine and norfluoxetine.

The present results were obtained in a study involving few patients, and the data should be supported with a larger number of patients and controls, preferably with repeated measurements. Although the question of cause or consequence remains unanswered, the present work is compatible with a possible immunological and endocrinological contribution to the cause of the depressive state. In this case, pharmacological treatment of depression may result in an enhanced immune competence, as indicated by increased NK cell activity. If indeed antidepressant drugs are capable of enhancing immune competence, their use would appear justified in individuals with compromised immune function, such as cancer.

Acknowledgements

The authors would like to express their deepest appreciation to the many patients who cooperated in the present study. The study was reported at the 40th Congress of Psychosomatic Medicine (Aomori: 1999).

References

Jozuka, H.: Panic attacks and serum IgE levels in depressive state. Clin Psychiat 1988; 25:87-91.

Jozuka, H.: T lymphocyte subsets in severe depressions. Teishin-Igaku 1988; 40:477-482.

Jozuka, H.: T lymphocyte subsets in panic disorders. Clin Psychiat 1989; 31:1336-1340.

Jozuka, H.: The immunological studies in anxiety and depressive state. Teishin-Igaku 1990; 42:599-605.

Jozuka, H.: Endogenous psychiatric disorders and immune responses. IMAGO 1993; 12:122-131.

Masek, K., Petrovicky, P., Sevcik, J., Zidek, Z., Frankova, D.: Past, present and future of psychoneuroimmunology. Toxicology 2000; 142:179-88.

Webster, J. I., Tonelli, L., Sternberg, E. M.: Neuroendocrine regulation of immunity. Annu Rev Immunol 2002; 20:125-63.

Raison, C. L., Miller, A.H.: The neuroimmunology of stress and depression. Semin Clin Neuropsychiatry 2001;6:277-94.

Sluzewska, A., Rybakowski, J., Bosmans, E., Sobieska, M., Berghmans, R., Maes, M., Wiktorowicz, K.: Indicators of immune

activation in severe depression. Psychiatry Res 1996;64:161-167.
Sluzewska, A.: Indicators of immune activation in depressed patients. Adv Exp Med Biol 1999;461:59-73.
Irwin, M.: Immune correlates of depression. Adv Exp Med Biol 1999;461:1-24.
Maes, M., Bosmans, E., Suy, E, Vandervorst C, DeJonckheere, C., Raus, J.: Immune disturbances during severe depression: upregulated expression of interleukin-2 receptors. Neuropsychobiology 1990-91;24:115-120.
Maes, M., Bonaccorso, S., Marino, V., Puzella, A., Pasquini, M., Biondi, M., Artini, M., Almerighi, C., Meltzer, H.: Treatment with interferon-alpha (IFN alpha) of hepatitis C patients induces lower serum dipeptidyl peptidase IV activity, which is related to IFN alpha-induced depressive and anxiety symptoms and immune activation. Mol Psychiatry 2001;6:475-480.
van West, D., Maes, M.: Activation of the inflammatory response system: A new look at the etiopathogenesis of severe depression. Neuroendocrinol Lett 1999;20:11-17.
Nishikaze, O.: Stress and clinical examinations. Clin Pathol 1994;42:321-330.
Nishikaze, O., Furuya, E.: Stress and anticortisols – 17-ketosteroid sulfate conjugate as a biomarker in time repair and recovery. J UOEH 1998;20:273-295.
Nishikaze, O., Furuya, E.: Healthy control: 17-KSSulfate. Science of Labor 1999;54:29-33.
Jozuka, H.: Psychoneuroimmunopathology. Nagoya: Marusen; 2000.
Goodyer, I.M., Herbert, J., Altham, P. M., Pearson, J., Secher, S. M., Shiers, H.M.: Adrenal secretion during severe depression in 8- to 16-year-olds, I. Altered diurnal rhythms in salivary cortisol and dehydroepiandrosterone (DHEA) at presentation. Psychol Med 1996;26:245-256.
Cruse, J. M., Lewis, R. E.: Atlas of Immunology. New York: CRC Press; 1998. p. 23-58, 185-206.

Osumi, K.: Natural killer cell activity. Clin Pathol 1982;45:299-304.

Baulieu, E. E.: Neurosteroids. Totowa: Humana Press; 1990.

Zung, W. W., Richards, C. B., Short, M. J.: Self-rating depression scale in an outpatient clinic. Further validation of the SDS. Arch Gen Psychiatry 1965;13:508-515.

Caldwell, C. L., Irwin, M., Lohr, J.: Reduced natural killer cell cytotoxicity in depression but not in schizophrenia. Biol Psychiatry 1991;30:1131-1138.

Irwin, M., Lacher, U., Caldwell, C. L.: Depression and reduced natural killer cytotoxicity: a longitudinal study of depressed patients and control subjects. Psychol Med 1992;22:1045-1050.

Mohl, P. C., Huang, L., Bowden, C., Fischbach, M., Vogtsberger, K., Talal, N.: Natural killer cell activity in severe depression. Am J Psychiatry 1987;144:1619.

Rook, A. H., Hooks, J. J., Quinnan, G. V., Lane, H. C., Manischewitz, J. F., Macher, A. M., Masur, H., Fauci, A. S., Djeu, J. Y.: Interleukin 2 enhances the natural killer cell activity of acquired immunodeficiency syndrome patients through a gamma-interferon-independent mechanism. J Immunol 1985, 134:1503-1507.

Weizman, R., Laor, N., Podliszewski, E., Notti, I., Djaldetti, M., Bessler, H.: Cytokine production in severe depressed patients before and after clomipramine treatment. Biol Psychiatry 1994;35:42-47.

Carson, W. E., Yu, H., Dierksheide, J., Pfeffer, K., Bouchard, P., Clark, R., Durbin, J., Baldwin, A. S., Peschon, J., Johnson, P. R., Ku, G., Baumann, H., Caligiuri, M. A.: A fatal cytokine-induced systemic inflammatory response reveals a critical role for NK cells. J Immunol 1999;162:4943-4951.

Maes, M., Capuron, L., Ravaud, A., Gualde, N., Bosmans, E., Egyed, B., Dantzer, R., Neveu, P. J.: Lowered serum dipeptidyl peptidase IV activity is associated with depressive symptoms and cytokine production in cancer patients receiving interleukin-2-based immunotherapy. Neuropsychopharma-

cology 2001;24:130-40.
Kathol, R. G.: Circannual rhythm and peak frequency of corticosteroid excretion: relationship to affective disorder. Psychiatr Med 1985;3:53-63.
Herman, J. P., Watson, S. J.: Stress regulation of mineralocorticoid receptor heteronuclear RNA in rat hippocampus. Brain Res 1995;677:243-249.
Stein, M., Miller, A., Tresman, R.: Depression and the immune system. In: Adel E, ed. Psychoneuroimmunology. New York: Academic Press, 1991.
Miller, A. H., Asnis, G. M., Lackner, C., Halbreich, U., Norin, A. J.: Depression, natural killer cell activity, and cortisol secretion. Biol Psychiatry 1991;29:878-886.
Loria, R. M., Padgett, D. A., Huynh, P. N.: Regulation of the immune response by dehydroepiandrosterone and its metabolites. J Endocrinol 1996;150:S209-S220.
Yamawaki, N., Takebayashi, M.: Steroid hormones and psychiatric symptoms. Current insights in neurological science, 1996.
Furuya, E., Maezawa, M., Nishikaze, O.: 17-KSSulfate as a biomarker in psychosocial stress. Clin Pathol 1998;46:529-537.
Wolkowitz, O. M., Reus, V. I., Roberts, E., Manfredi, F., Chan, T., Raum, W. J., Ormiston, S., Johnson, R., Canick, J., Brizendine, L., Weingartner, H.: Dehydroepiandrosterone (DHEA) treatment of depression. Biol Psychiatry 1997;41:311-318.
Frank, M. G., Hendricks, S. E., Johnson, D. R., Wieseler, J. L., Burke, W. J.: Antidepressants augment natural killer cell activity: in vivo and in vitro. Neuropsychobiology 1999;39:18-24.
Helgason, C. M., Frank, J. L., Johnson, D. R., Frank, M. G., Hendricks, S. E.: The effects of St. John's Wort (Hypericum perforatum) on NK cell activity in vitro. Immunopharmacology 2000;46:247-251.

Table 1: Measurements of parameters in healthy controls and in patients with severe depression

Healthy controls (n = 10)	Depressed patients (n = 17)	
26.4 ± 17.3	7.5 ± 2.5 **	NK cell activity (%)
344 ± 98	542 ± 111 **	IL-2 (pg/ml)
12.3 ± 3.8	7.1 ± 4.5 *	Cortisol (μg/dl)
5.6 ± 1.5	3.3 ± 0.8 **	DHEA (mg/ml)
1116 ± 452	1621 ± 818	DHEA-S (mg/ml)
32 ± 7	55 ± 3 **	SDS score

Values represent mean ± SD. * $p < 0.05$; ** $p < 0.01$ when compared to controls. DHEA: Dehydroepiandrosterone; SDS: Zunf Self-Rating Depression Scale

> "The results revealed that it would be important to start treating depression by the use of SSRIs and DHEA including intensive psychotherapy to prevent cancers."

Practical Applications of Psychoneuroimmunopathology

The authors will explain several clinical experiences using PNIP.

- Malignant Neoplasm
- Allergic Diseases
- Chronic Fatigue Syndrome
- Coronary Heart Diseases

First, the authors will discuss eight patients in the terminal stage of cancer. Their medical specialists from famous medical schools have already informed all the patients.

I. Practical Application in Cancer: Patients Suffering from Malignant Neoplasm who were Treated Using PNIP

The number of patients suffering from malignant neoplasms (cancers) has increased rapidly over the previous 30 years. Because of the increase in patients, treatment methods are increasing and being developed daily.

The increase in the number of treatable patients is similar to the increase in the number of untreatable patients. Therefore, a large amount of studies and research on the treatment of malignant neoplasms has been performed, particularly on non-surgical treatments. Patients who are considered incurable by contemporary methods have been casually abandoned by medicine. Therefore, they had no choice but to enter a hospice. As a result, the importance of integrative medicine and/or holistic medicine has greatly increased.

Flv.: Fluvoxamine; AT: Autogenic Training; Psy. Anal.: Simple Psychoanalysis; Gly.: Glycyrrhizinic acid; DHEA: dehydroepiandrosterone; Mlp.: Milnacipran; Met.: metastasis; Dulox.: Duloxetine

Age	Sex	Diagnosis	Medications	Main-Psychotherapy	Added Life Span
33	M	Heart Myosarcoma	Dosulepine	Laughter therapy	3 months
42	F	Breast Cancer and Virchow Ly	Flv.	AT and Psy. Anal.	more than 10 years
52	F	C-viral Hepatoma	Flv. Gly. acid DAEA	Daseinsanalysis	more than 10 years
68	F	C-viral Hepatomamet. brain	Mlp. Gly. DHEA	Daseinsanalysis	more than 10 years
55	F	C-viral Hepatoma met. Brain, bones, etc.	Flv. Gly. acid DHEA	Laughter therapy	8 months
53	F	C-viral Hepatoma, Cirrhosis	Flv. Gly. DHEA	Laughter Therapy and Daseinsanalysis	more than 10 years
48	F	Myosarcoma uterus, lung, brain	Flv.	Daseinsanalysis	3.5 years
62	F	C-viral Hepatoma	Flv. Gly.	Simple psychotherapy	5.3 years
54	F	C-viral Hepatoma(3x2 cm)	Flv. Dulox.Gly.	Laughter Therapy	15 years
63	M	Nonviral hepatoma	Flv.	Daseinsanalysis	15 years
68	F	Uterus Carc.	Flv.	Daseinsanalysis	15 years
43	M	Malignant Lymphoma	Flv.	Laughter therapy	10 years

Table 1. Patients Suffering from Malignant Neoplasms in Organs (all clients had been informed by famous specialists that no method of treatment was available.)

It is common for incurable and/or untreatable patients to be informed that their cancer is terminal. They are told, "You will pass away in exactly three months, so you must spend quality time with your family in your remaining days. There is no more treatment available for you in the world."

Such information usually causes patients to fall into depression and also reduces their immune responses against cancers. Bartrop, RW has previously reported on this problem. [32]

A group of patients wanted to attempt other treatments, and by chance, they visited us to try PNIP treatments as their last hope. Their profiles, diagnoses, and treatment methods using PNIP (including medication and psychotherapy) are shown in **Table 1**.

"Regression of Hepatocellular Carcinoma During Psychoneuroimmunopathological Therapy – A case Report" From Jozuka, H: Current Medical Research and Opinion vol. 19, No. 1, 2003©

Introduction

The authors will illustrate the basic method of PNIP treatment through a typical case of terminal stage cancer.

Recently, the development of psychoneuroimmunology and psycho-oncology has changed the approach to patients suffering from advanced stage cancer and has even affected the philosophy of medicine. [1] At the present time, advanced stage cancer patients do not wait patiently for death but want to live as long and as fully as possible. Doctors tend to examine specific physical organs but tend to ignore the importance of the patient's mind. Most doctors believe that patients suffering from advanced stage cancer with approximately one to three months to live should spend this time enjoying their family. Often no anticancer treatment is prescribed for these patients, and no psychological/psychiatric support is provided. Only analgesics are given routinely. Therefore, only patients who suffer from cancer and subsequently become depressed visit psychiatrists to seek mental support.

A patient with hepatocellular carcinoma who became depressed was treated by us using a psychoneuroimmunopathological approach founded on the idea that ill health is based on psychopathological problems that lead to various clinical abnormalities such as psychological, neurological, endocrinological and immunological changes.

Materials and Methods
Patient

The 52-year-old female patient was sociable, obliging, cheerful, and intelligent with a cyclothymic personality; she worked as a beautician. Because her husband was a chronic gambler, she was obliged to provide for the entire household, and this situation caused her constant stress. In addition, she had never been pregnant, which caused her identity problems as a woman and led to a continuous state of conflict. She visited her physician for a common cold, and after biochemical tests of peripheral blood cells, the diagnosis of hepatitis C was determined.

After several months, her general fatigue had increased, and she decided to visit the largest hospital in the town as suggested by her physician. The results of biochemical and peripheral blood cells and a CT scan of her abdomen indicated that the development of her hepatitis C was too severe to treat. She visited many doctors in hospitals and other physicians who gave her the same answer. Her condition worsened, she became depressed and she even considered suicide. She could not go on working as a beautician and became bedridden. A previous client from the beauty parlor suggested that she visit our clinic where psychoneuroimmunopathological approaches were used.

When she came to our clinic, she was suffering from sleep disturbance (early morning waking), depressive mood and severe irritation, suicidal ideation, reduction of activity, severe general fatigue, abdominal fullness, general itching of the skin, and cancer phobia. Her self-rating depression scale (SDS) score (Zung) was 78. Her features were drawn, and her skin was edematous and dark brown colored; severe abdominal edema was also observed.

The biochemical examinations showed destruction and fibrosis of liver cells, increase of the tumor marker a-fetoprotein, reduction of repair ability (reduction of dehydroepiandrosterone [DHEA] and cortisol) and increased immune responses. From these results and a CT-scan, she was diagnosed as having hepatocellular carcinoma and was suffering from severe depression according to DSM-IV criteria.

Methods

The patient was treated on an outpatient basis. Markers of liver, immunological, and endocrinological functions were measured in the serum regularly for the first month and then monthly. Treatment consisted of daily music therapy and aromatherapy for one to two hours before and after a daily injection of glycyrrhizinic acid, daily laughter therapy for approximately half an hour and weekly psychotherapy (supportive and psychopathological analytic approach). The saponin, glycyrrhizinic acid (60 ml/day), the selective serotonin reuptake inhibitor (SSRI) antidepressant, fluvoxamine (50 mg/day), the anxiolytic, flutoprazepam (2 mg/day), the sedative, lormetazoram (1 mg/day) and DHEA (50 mg/day) were administered.

Results

The first biochemical tests (July 1999) showed reduced liver function (aspartate aminotransferase (AST), alanine aminotransferase (ALT), lactate deshydrogenase (LDH), alkaline phosphatase (ALP), g-glutamyl transpeptidase (g-GTP)), high levels of hyaluronic acid (HA), a-fetoprotein, and low levels of cortisol and DHEA. (Table 1) Immunologically, increased natural killer (NK) cell activity and interleukin (IL)-2, IL-6, IL-12 and interferon (IFN-g) were observed. (Table 1) The patient was depressed (score of 78 on the SDS) (Table 1) and irritable. After two weeks of treatment, her depressive mood and irritation gradually decreased; however, high levels of HA (464.3 ng/ml) and a-fetoprotein (104.3 ng/ml) persisted, and liver function (AST and ALT) was still reduced. After approximately a month, although her anxiety and fear of death had been increasing, she began to smile, and her NK cell activity and IL-6 started to decrease, whereas there was a major increase in her IL-2 levels. After 3 months of treatment (Table 1), her liver function (AST, ALT) was improved and her HA was increased; although a-fetoprotein remained high, NK cell activity showed a decrease and IL-12 displayed an increase. The patient was still depressed with suicidal ideation. After 6 months, the abdominal edema was reduced, and she had a good appetite. At that time, the levels of AST, ALT and a-fetoprotein were close to normal, whereas the levels of HA were increased and NK cell activity had increased slightly. At that time, the dose of fluvoxamine was increased to 100 mg/day. A month later, all of the biochemical tests showed values close to normal, except for HA (763 ng/ml). It was concluded that she no longer suffered from cancer. She had also recovered from her depression.

After 9 months of treatment (Table 1), all of her biochemical values were close to normal. Two and a half years later, all of her values continued to be normal. Glycyrrhizinic acid (60 ml/day), fluvoxamine (100 mg/day), and DHEA (50 mg/day) are still administered and psychotherapy is continuing.

Discussion

It is a common belief that psychopathological problems lead to a reduction of immunological capacity, and consequently, patients are more susceptible to infections such as hepatoma C virus, which can evolve into carcinogenesis. [2]

Hepatoma C virus is an RNA virus and, unlike hepatoma B virus, it is not incorporated into the host genome. [3] The tumor may evolve from fibrogenesis rather than from the hepatoma C virus infection itself because cirrhosis is already established in most cases. [3] In the present case, cirrhosis was absent because HA levels were very variable. In the case reported here, immunological measurements of NK cell activity, IL-2, IL-6, IL-12 and IFN-g were performed. NK cells are lymphoid cells of the natural immune system that express cytotoxicity against various nucleated cells including tumor cells and virus-infected cells. [4] NK cell activity in the present case showed high levels, at entry and again at six months. IL-2 promotes NK cell growth and potentates the cytolytic action of NK cells through the generation of lymphokine-activated killer cells (LAK). [4] In addition, IL-2 promotes the improved responsiveness of immature bone marrow cells to other cytokines. [4] The levels of IL-2 were high throughout the first six months. IL-6 is the main factor that activates B-lymphocytes, and it acts in concert with other cytokines to promote the growth of early hematopoietic stem cells. [4] Although the level of IL-6 was very high (20.4 pg/ml) at entry, its levels decreased during treatment. IL-12 serves as a natural killer cell stimulatory factor by facilitating NK cell and LAK cell lytic action. IL-12 may act synergistically with IL-2 to increase responses by cytotoxic lymphocytes. [4] IFN-g, called Type II interferon in the past, is formed mainly by T-lymphocytes stimulated by antigens or mitogens and by NK cells. Although the ability of interferon to prevent the infection of non-infected cells is species-specific, it is not virus-specific. All viruses are subject to its inhibitory action. Interferon induces the formation of a second inhibitory protein that prevents viral mRNA translation. [4] These data suggest that the treatment used here contributes immunologically to the destruction of the cancer, particularly through the action of NK cells and IL-12 and secondarily through IL-2 and IFN-g. Currently, the treatment of hepatocellular carcinoma is primarily immunological with IFN-g through both a direct effect of IFN-g and by its secondary effect of increasing NK cell activity, which is thought to destroy cancer cells.

[5] Moreover, treatment with Il-12, which is still at an experimental level, promises to be very effective in treating cancers. [6]

As mentioned above, the high level of NK cell activity was likely due to hepatocellular carcinoma. However, a reduction of NK cell activity and an increase of IL-2 have been observed in severe depression. [7] With treatment, an increase in immunological responses such as NK cell activity, IL-2, IL-6, IL-12 and IFN-g can be expected, in addition to an increase of DHEA and cortisol. [7,8] It appears that the increase of NK cell activity and IL-2 leads to the formation and increase of IFN-g. [5] However, the levels of IL-6 and IL-12 were also observed. These responses occur before responses of cytotoxic T cell and virus-specific immune reactions. [5] Therefore, primarily activated NK cells destroy virus-infected cells, and IFN-g protects non-infected cells. These reactions prevent the spread of viral infection. [5] Depression is associated with a decrease in immune reactions, [7] and the permanent stress state of the present case led to depression with a consequently reduced immune response. Laughter therapy is believed to promote enhancement of immunological competences such as NK cell activity. [9] Some studies have shown that the levels of cAMP are enhanced by stress, and this increase in cAMP decreases the levels of IFN-g and IL-2. [2] The psychotherapy and laughter therapy used here have led to opposite results. Many studies report that psychotherapy and relaxation therapy may increase NK cell activity and IL-2 levels. [10-19] In addition, relaxation by use of -wave music and aromatherapy has been shown to enhance immunological responses. [20-22]

Recently, increases in NK cell activity by several antidepressants have been reported by Franck et al. [23], and more specifically, the same findings have been found with the use of fluvoxamine. [24] The natural phenomena of the reduction in NK cell activity and the increase in IL-2 observed in depression are followed by an increase in NK cell activity and a reduction in IL-2 during recovery from depression. [7] Therefore, these immunological changes might be caused by the effect of fluvoxamine used in the present work.

Glycyrrhizin is a saponine ingredient of kanzo, a traditional Chinese medicine. The effects of glycyrrhizin are mainly anti-inflammatory, anti-allergic, and immunomodulatory, and they cause the suppression of virus-proliferation. [25] In patients suffering from chronic hepatitis, ALT levels are reduced by glycyrrhizin, and with long-term injections of glycyrrhizinic acid (2 to 16 years), carcinogenesis can be prevented in patients suffering from hepatitis C. [26] Glycyrrhizinic acid has also been suggested to increase IFN-g, IL-2, IL-6 and Il-12. [27] Therefore, in the present study, it is possible that glycyrrhizinic acid might have contributed to the regression of hepatoma C.

An immunological role has been attributed to DHEA by Nishikaze [28] and Nishikaze and Furuya. [29-30] DHEA promotes the activation of immune responses such as synthesis and the increase of cytokines. [31] Because DHEA is produced in the brain, its levels are influenced by psychosomatic phenomena. The roles of DHEA are suggested to be cellular repair and recovery. [7] In the present study, the initial DHEA levels were very low, but the administration of DHEA and, with recovery, the endogenous levels, may have led to the activation of immune responses.

Four other patients suffering from hepatocellular carcinoma from April 1993 to December 1996 were treated in a manner similar to the case described here and showed the same regression of their disease. However, there are not yet enough cases available to analyze the results statistically.

In conclusion, the patients treated by psychotherapy, antidepressants, glycyrrhizinic acid and DHEA according to the concept of psychoneuroimmunopathology recovered from hepatocellular carcinoma and have lived for more than five years without any problems or abnormalities.

Acknowledgment

The authors are grateful to Professor Hiroshi Yoshizawa, a specialist in hepatology, for his suggestions in diagnoses and treatment.

References

Jozuka, H.: Psychoneuroimmunopathology. Nagoya, Maruzen, 2000.

Yata, J.: Immunology for Clinicians - "Stress and Immunomechanism". Nippon Ijishinposha, 1999, pp 178.

Yoshisawa, H., Ino, S.: Viral hepatitis - Diagnosis and prevention. Bunko-Do, Tokyo, 1999.

Cruse, J. M., Lewis, R. E.: Atlas of Immunology, CRC Press, New York, 1998, pp 23-58, 185-206.

Katsura, Y., Ohbi, T.: Immunology. Kinphodo, 1995, pp 54-56.

Barajas, M., Mazzolini, G., Genove, G., Bilbao, R., Narvaiza, I., Schmitz, V., Sangro, B., Melero, I., Qian, C., Prieto, J.: Gene therapy of orthotopic hepatocellular carcinoma in rats using adenovirus coding for interleukin 12. Hepatology 2001;33:52-61.

Jozuka, H., Jozuka, E., Takeuchi, S., Suzuki, M., Takumi, K., Tokuhiro, C., Saito, M.: Psychoneuroendocrinological study in severe depressions. Clin Psychiat 2000;6:599-604.

Unai, Y.: The studies on psychological phenomena and immunological mechanisms: especially relationships depression. J Showa Medical Univ 1998;58:18-29.

Itami, J. Noboru, M., Teshima, H.: Laughing and immune responses. J Psychosom 1994;34:565-571.

Green, S.: Mind-body research in psychooncology. Adv Mind Body Med:1999;236-244.

Newport, D. J., Nemeroff, C. B.: Assessment and treatment of depression in the cancer patient. J Psychosom Res 1998;45:215-237.

Lekander, M., Furst, C. J., Rotstein, S., Hursti, T. J., Fredrikson, M.: Immune effects of relaxation during chemotherapy for ovarian cancer. Psychother Psychosom 1997;66:185-191.

de Vries, M. J., Schilder, J. N., Mulder, C. L., Vrancken, A. M., Remie, M., Garssen, B.: Phase II study of psychotherapeutic intervention in advanced cancer. Psychooncology 1997;6:129-137.

van der Pompe, G., Antoni, M., Visser, A., Garssen, B.: Adjustment to breast cancer: the psychobiological effects of psychosocial interventions. Patient Educ Couns 1996;28:209-219.

van der Pompe ,G., Duivenvoorden, H. J., Antoni, M. H., Visser,

A., Heijnen, C. J.: Effectiveness of a short-term group psychotherapy program on endocrine and immune function in breast cancer patients: an exploratory study. J Psychosom Res 1997;42:453-466.

Rood, Y. R., Bogaards, M., Goulmy, E., Houwelingen, H. C.: The effects of stress and relaxation on the in vitro immune response in man: a meta-analytic study. J Behav Med 1993;16:163-181.

Fawzy, F. I., Kemeny, M. E., Fawzy, N. W., Elashoff, R., Morton, D., Cousins, N., Fahey, J. L.: A structured psychiatric intervention for cancer patients. II. Changes over time in immunological measures. Arch Gen Psychiatry 1990;47:729-735.

Udelman, D. L., Udelman, H. D.: A preliminary report on antidepressant therapy and its effects on hope and immunity. Soc Sci Med 1985;20:1069-1072.

Jozuka, H., Saito, M.: Cancer, Stress and Immunology Vol. 2C: Changes of NK cell activities in the patient of progressive cancer. J Psychosom 1999;39:134.

Kubota, S.: The scientific of music therapy. J Japanese Biomusic Association 2000;18:20.

Kubota, S., Hasegawa, Y.: Before and after changes of NK cell activities and other characteristics in old persons. J Japanese Biomusic Association 1999;17:183-187.

Noda, R.: Palliative Care; Ideations and Methods of Nursing; The Points of View as Total Care for Patients of Cancers. Music Therapy; The Significance of Palliative Care. The Music and Exercise Therapy. J Clin Nursing 1996;22:2067-2072.

Frank, M. G., Hendricks, S. E., Johnson, D. R., Wieseler, J. L., Burke, W. J.: Antidepressants augment natural killer cell activity: in vivo and in vitro. Neuropsychobiology 1999;39:18-24.

Ballin, A., Gershon, V., Tanay, A., Brener, J., Weizman, A., Meytes, D.: The antidepressant fluvoxamine increases natural killer cell counts in cancer patients. Isr J Med Sci 1997;

33:720-723.
Okita, K.: Cirrhosis and Hepatocellular Cancer (Diagnoses and Treatment). Nankodo, 2000.
Arase, Y., Ikeda, K., Murashima, N., Chayama, K, Tsubota, A., Koida, I., Suzuki, Y., Saitoh, S., Kobayashi, M., Kumada, H.: The long term efficacy of glycyrrhizin in chronic hepatitis C patients. Cancer 1997;79:1494-1500.
Abe, N., Ebina, T., Ishida, N.: Interferon induction by glycyrrhizin and glycyrrhetinic acid in mice. Microbiol Immunol 1982;26:535-539.
Nishikaze, O.: Stress and clinical examinations. J Clin Pathol 1994;42:321-330.
Nishikaze, O., Furuya, E.: Stress and anticortisols – 17-ketosteroid sulfate conjugate as a biomarker in tissue repair and recovery. J UOEH 1998;20:273-295.
Nishikaze, O., Furuya, E.: Healthy control: 17-KS-Sulfate. Science of Labor 1999;54:29-33.
Loria, R. M., Padgett, D. A., Huynh, P. N.: Regulation of the immune response by dehydroepiandrosterone and its metabolites. J Endocrinol 1996;150:S209-S220.
Bartrop, R. W., et al.: Depressed lymphocyte function after bereavement. Lancet 1:834, 1977.

Explanation of the Table

The values are the scores of the self-rating depression scale (SDS) and the serum measurements of biochemical examinations at the beginning when the diagnosis of hepatocellular carcinoma was established. AST = aspartate aminotransferase, ALT = alanine aminotransferase, LDH = lactate dehydrogenase, ALP = alkaline phosphatase, g-GTP = g-glutamyl transpeptidase, HA = hyaluronic acid, DHEA = dehydroepian (July 1999) before treatment and at the 3rd, 6th and 9th months when the condition of the patient was considered to be drosterone, DHEA-S = dehydroepiandrosterone-sulphate, NK = natural killer, IL = interleukine, IFN-g = interferon. nd = not determined.

Table 1. Biochemical evaluations before and during treatment

Normal values	1st examinati on July 1999	Examinati on after 3rd month of treatment	Examinati on after 6th month of treatment	Examinati on after 9th month of treatment	
< 50	78	66	38	32	AST (IU/l)
1-40	229	80	51	38	ALT (IU/l)
1-35	331	84	42	39	LDH (IU/l)
100-400	714	596	508	460	ALP (IU/l)
80-280	321	222	243	322	γ-GTP (IU/l)
0-45	293	145	51	42	HA (ng/ml)
< 50	171.1	489.4	813.3	109.8	α-fetoprotein (ng/ml)
< 20	80.3	62.3	38	9.2	Cortisol (μg/dl)
2-20	1.8	1.8	6.2	18	DHEA ng/ml
1.0-10.0	1	4.6	5.5	2.2	DHEA-S (ng/ml)
800-4600	70	856	2640	693	NK cell activity (%)
5-25	33.5	7.1	31.1	10.1	IL-2 productivity (pg/ml)
220-630	497	405	660	248	IL-6 (pg/ml)
< 20	20.4	1.8	nd	4.2	IL-12 (pg/ml)
10-15	60.8	93.7	nd	252	IFN-γ (IU/ml)
< 0.1	0.32	0.1	nd	0.1	

Values are the scores of self-rating depression scale (SDS) and the serum measurements of biochemical examinations at the beginning when the diagnosis of hepatocellular carcinoma was established remitted. AST = aspartate aminotransferase, ALT = alanine aminotransferase, LDH = lactate dehydrogenase, ALP = alkaline phosphatase, g-GTP = g-glutamyl transpeptidase, HA = hyaluronic acid, DHEA = dehydroepian (July 1999) before treatment and at 3rd, 6th and 9th months when the condition of the patient was considered to be drosterone, DHEA-S = dehydroepiandrosterone-sulphate, NK = natural killer, IL = interleukine, IFN-g = interferon. nd = not determined.

The Details of the Actual Treatment of a Typical Case shown in Table 1

Several top liver cancer specialists in universities had already informed the patient of her terminal state. Subsequently, she became severely depressed to the point of attempting suicide. She also suffered from insomnia.

After holistic medical examinations using PNIP, she was informed that the treatment would be performed only in an attempt to prolong her life. She immediately agreed to receive any treatment to live longer.

A. Stage One
At the beginning of the treatment, her immune abilities were low but still within hope of recovery. She said, "Upon receiving the injections, I felt as if the whole agony subsided, so I decided to fight against the disease."

B. Stage Two
As the therapist-patient relationship deepened, the psychoanalytic approach was used. They began by talking about her phenomenological past and her lifestyle. She began to feel separate from her disease as she talked about her past from the time she was approximately 10 years old until her adolescence, why she married her husband and how her lifestyle changed, until the development of the disease. Then, her immune responses gradually increased.

C. Stages Three and Four
Her resistance against the disease grew stronger, and she felt it was actually separate from her. She and the authors kept fighting against it together. At the time, her immune responses against her disease showed the consistently highest levels until the disappearance of her disease.

D. Stage Five
Finally, upon seeing the results of the tests, she was surprised, and even shouted: "Our enemy is gone! We won!"

Thus, the entire course of treatment using PNIP finished successfully. From then on, her treatment consisted of maintenance against relapse. She will receive periodic psychotherapy, oral medications, and injections. Even if her PNIP treatment ends, she must continue the maintenance plan until complete remission, defined in PNIP as 10 additional years of life instead of the common definition of 5 years.

Practical Psychotherapy Based on Daseinsanalysis

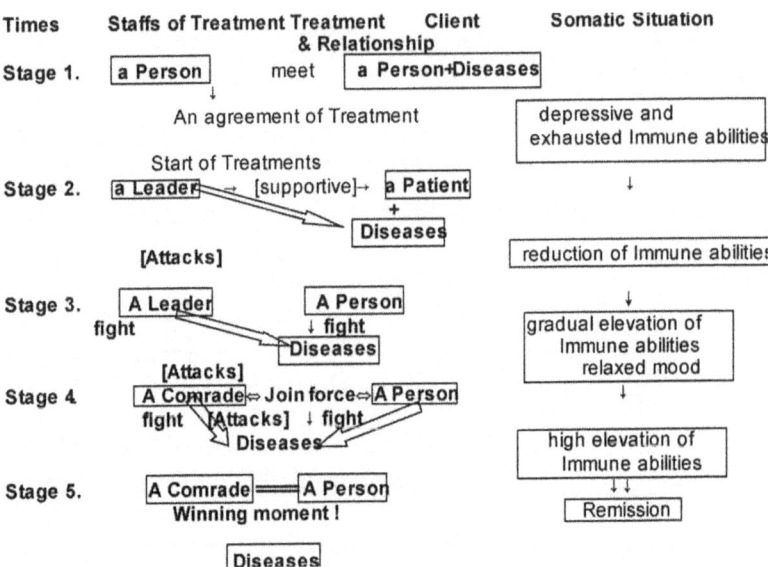

Figure 1. Practical Psychotherapy based on 'Daseinsanalysis'

Case of a Patient who Suffered from Breast Cancer Metastasized to Her Virchow Lymph Node

The authors encountered a rare case of a woman suffering from breast cancer that had metastasized to her Virchow lymph node. The details of the case will be introduced. More than 10 years later, she is still living and enjoying life with her new husband.

Introduction

Many reports and studies of patients suffering from breast cancer are available. Many of these studies are usually studies of clients suffering from metastasized cancers. Therefore, such studies consider not only how to live longer with treatments but also how to live with cancer. In other words, they are studies based on terminal care.

However, even the clients who are in a terminal stage and receiving terminal care have an ambivalent idea that allows them to hope to live as long as possible even though they are receiving therapy on how to die peacefully.

Usually clients in the terminal stage receive only terminal care, which focuses on how to die rather than on how to live.

Recently, several clients who had been informed that they were in a terminal stage of cancer visited the author's clinic to receive additional treatments, and they have continued to live. Many clients hope for recovery from terminal and metastasized cancers. It is a fundamental idea in humans to hope to live and never to die.

Consequently, the authors and staffs always try to contact and treat clients suffering from cancer to help them live as long as they hope to, even though they have been informed that their life will end within several weeks or months. Fortunately, although the authors have been treating so-called terminal clients for more than 15 years, only one client, who had myocardial sarcoma at the center of the heart muscle when he came for treatment, died three months after visiting the authors.

The following is a description of a typical case study of a prospective PNIP client. The client, who was informed that she was in a terminal stage of cancer, visited the author and has continued to live for more ten years. This case of a typical client who received PNIP treatment and approaches is described as follows:

Explanation of the Case
The patient was a 42-year-old female who was a desk worker in a small contracting company. The woman was quick-tempered and sociable with a variable temper (cycloid personality).

Diagnosis:
Breast cancer metastasized to Virchow lymph node after surgery. Depressive state (clinically diagnosed not as bipolar disorder but as severe depression by the DSM-III-R).

Course of Illness
Since the sudden death of her husband from a malignant brain tumor, the patient has been undergoing thorough examinations once every three months. No abnormal findings had been observed for three years, but three weeks after the usual examination she noticed a lump in her left breast. She visited a surgeon in the large central hospital. She was diagnosed as suffering from breast cancer and thus underwent surgery. Although the operation was successful, after a week she noticed swelling and pain in the area around her left clavicle. This indicated metastasis to the Virchow lymph node. The surgeon informed her that she had approximately three months to live. A second operation was performed immediately to extirpate her Virchow lymph node.

Although she was depressed, she fervently hoped to live. She was diagnosed as suffering from severe depression and was moved into a psychiatric ward in the same hospital.

She discharged herself from the hospital despite opposition from a psychiatrist and promptly visited the author's clinic. Although anticancer agents were prescribed, she refused to take them.

The psychosomatic findings at her first consultation were confusion with crying, depressive mood without activity, irritation, general fatigue, and sleep disturbance.

In chemical examinations, her natural killer cell activity and serum cortisol showed severely low levels as follows: her natural killer cell activity was 4.5 % and her serum cortisol was 1.2 g/dl.

Treatment Plan

The authors and staff set up the following treatment plan:
SSRI (Fluvoxamine 100 mg/2/day) was prescribed to improve her mental symptoms and to elevate her natural killer cell activity.

For several months, she underwent supportive psychotherapy until there was an improvement in her depressive state. She then underwent psychopathological therapies including autogenic training, -wave music therapy, and aromatherapy. (She could not undergo complete Daseinsanalysis).

She had to agree to undergo thorough examinations by her surgeon.

Course of Treatment:

The course of treatment, which included changing stressors, variations in natural killer cell activity, and serum cortisol values, is explained in the description.

From her first consultation, she received treatments regularly once a week.

She began by complaining about her life history. She said, "Since losing my husband, I have been raising my two children by myself, with no one to give me support. I thought it was my duty to live just because of my children, so I have been undergoing thorough examinations regularly because my husband died from a malignant brain tumor. However, no surgeon found my breast cancer. I discovered it. Furthermore, it was me who discovered the metastasis to the lymph node, although I had been repeatedly examined. What a strange phenomenon has occurred! Finally, because I did not believe in my surgeon, I decided to visit your clinic to receive holistic medical treatment. I am sorry but I still do not have any faith in your treatments either. I will be able to believe you if I am still living when my children grow up and enter university."

Following her explanation of her inner world and psycho-pathogenic life history, her natural killer cell activity gradually increased. Six months after her first visit, her natural killer cell activity was 10.2 % and her serum cortisol level was 5.3 g/dl. At the time, no metastasis was found in the regular examinations.

She decided to work part-time in an office. The office was not in a big company; consequently, she was not very busy. She was not tired because her boss was gentle with her and did not give her hard work.

After a year, her natural killer cell activity was 14.0 % and her serum cortisol was 8.1 g/dl (which are similar to the levels of a healthy person). Moreover, no malignant metastasized lesion was observed anywhere in her body. She began to believe more and more in the treatment and became friendly with the clinic stuff.

Her boss invited her to dinner in recognition of her progress in overcoming her health problems, but unfortunately, her boss raped her just as she was leaving.

The next day she visited the clinic and the usual parameters were measured. Her natural killer cell activity was 7.4 % and her serum cortisol was 5.1 g/dl. She was scared of a recurrence of the cancer and thus underwent thorough examinations at several hospitals. There were no abnormal findings.

Naturally, she decided to quit her office job and to concentrate on her treatments.

In psychotherapy, she explained her deep inner life history and the many problems she had encountered in the past. She seemed to be completely transformed by catharsis after two years of visiting the clinic. At the time, her natural killer cell activity was 24.5 % and her serum cortisol was 10.0 g/dl.

Seven years later, she works in another office in a major company. Her natural killer cell activity and serum cortisol are very similar to the above reading. Furthermore, no malignant findings have been observed during thorough examinations for approximately seven years.

She continues to visit the clinic to receive counseling, aromatherapy, and music therapy every week.

She sometimes visits the clinic with her new partner. Her daughter is about to get married, and her son will be joining a major company next year.

Additionally, she has not menstruated in a month, and her partner, who has not had any children of his own, hopes that she is pregnant.

She said, "It is a pleasure but also shameful to be a mother of a baby and a grandmother of my daughter's baby, but, I am deeply happy. I will visit you forever."

To this day, neither of her parameters has decreased.

Discussion and Conclusion

Breast cancer metastasized to the Virchow lymph node was described. There is great danger of general metastasis in such a situation. It would not have been surprising to find metastasized lesions anywhere in her body, but the client who suffered from this malignant cancer has been living for more than seven years.

On her first visit to the clinic, the client was in the "exhausted stage" of the Stress Theory, having undergone two operations and psychic trauma "handed out" by the surgeon. In such a situation, both parameters likely showed the lowest possible levels for a living person.

It is thought that these phenomena explained a reduction in psychosomatic energy. For the client in such a situation, the supportive psychotherapy and SSRI were so effective that both parameters gradually increased. When her boss raped her, her psychosomatic situation was not able to recover or confront the occurrence; both parameters showed severe reductions.

Fortunately, because she had been undergoing psychotherapies and taking Fluvoxamine regularly, her natural killer cell activity and serum cortisol elevated very quickly. Although the rape would cause her severe psychic trauma, both of her parameters increased again because of the support she received from her two children, her psychologist, her psychiatrist, etc. Most likely her immediate decision to quit the part-time office job was helped by the fact that she had many supporters.

From then on, she began to realize the importance of human relationships to the improvement of her general state of mind. She progressed in psychotherapy, and the levels of her natural killer cell activity and serum cortisol increased to higher levels. Moreover, no malignant lesions have been observed anywhere in her body despite the fact that she never took any anti-cancer agents.

From these observations, we can conclude that psychoneuroimmunopathological treatments can play an extremely important role in the improvement and recuperation from cancer.

It is thought that the woman's energy to confront her cancer came from her determination to bring up her two children. Her two children have now grown up and graduated from university. Her daughter is about to marry. Her son is about to leave home and begin working in a large company in another town. It will therefore be important for her to be under closer observation from now on. Fortunately, there is no doubt that her new husband will help elevate and/or keep her natural killer cell activity and serum cortisol at ordinary levels.

References
The references are the same as mentioned before.

Practical Application of PNIP in Allergic Diseases
Introduction
Allergic diseases have been thought to occur because of the presence of allergens. Thus, it has been assumed that allergic reactions never occur without large amounts of allergens. Furthermore, it is believed that allergic reactions are always found in persons who have a congenital allergic constitution. It is also believed that allergic reactions occur only as peripheral responses in human beings. The idea that allergic reactions relate to brain phenomena has been denied by most allergologists until today. In fact, pollen information is reported in newspapers and television news programs every day for people suffering from pollen allergies because people commonly believe that allergic diseases develop based on the quantity of pollen they are exposed to.

On the one hand, although many people show low IgE levels, they have in fact been suffering from allergic rhinitis. On the other hand, many people show high IgE levels but have never suffered from any allergic diseases.

Furthermore, the authors explain that catharsis, including relaxation, reduced IgE values in healthy people.

Based on these observations, it will be important to treat allergic diseases using psychopathological therapies. From this point of view, an interesting and typical case will be described below.

Additionally, the authors have treated many allergic clients for more than 20 years based on psychoneuroimmunopathology. Many cases have received psychopathological treatment including pathogeneses through the observation of endocrino-immune parameters.

Some Clients Who Suffered from Allergic Diseases
The author would like to present some clients who suffered from allergic disease. They were informed by the specialist, "Your disease can never be treated even with high doses of corticosteroid hormones such as Prednisolone and Betamethazone. They might provide relief for a short time but will just make it worse afterwards." Finally, they were told that their diseases were serious and incurable.

When the clients found out that they had a type of psychosomatic disease, they came to the authors for treatment.

Table 1. Patients suffering from Allergic Diseases
(M: male, F: female)

Age	Sex	Diagnosis	Treatments	IgE RIST level before treatment	Interval	IgE RIST level after (during) treatment
3.8	M	Atopic Dermatitis	Play Therapy	335,000 IU/ml	6 years	826 IU/ml
3.5	M	Bronchial Asthma	Play Therapy	7,2050 IU/ml	6 years	389 IU/ml
9.6	F	Bronchial Asthma	Play and Art Therapy	15,280 1U/ml	9 years	12 IU/ml
10.8	F	Bronchial Asthma	Play and Art Therapy	7,250 IU/ml	6 years	380 IU/ml
15.2	M	Atopic Dermatitis	Play and Art Therapy	20,900 IU/ml	8 years	450 IU/ml
19.8	M	Atopic Dermatitis	Dasein analysis	9,000 IU/ml	6 years	3,200 IU/ml
24.4	M	Atopic Dermatitis	Dasein analysis	6,000 IU/ml	8 years	3,250 IU/ml

(All clients had been rejected by famous specialists)

Description of a Typical Case
Here a typical case using PNIP will be described.

Case
The client was a 4-year-old male.

Diagnosis
The client was suffering from severe allergic dermatitis, commonly called atopic dermatitis (general inflammatory dermatitis except for the scalp).

Course of the Illness
Beginning at 2 years of age, a slight indication of atopic dermatitis began to be observed in the client. At the time, inflammatory changes were limited to the joints. At the rebellious stage of 3 years old, his dermatitis spread over his entire body, accompanied by intolerable itching. His mother took him to a dermatology department in a hospital. At the first hospital, he was given ointment containing corticosteroid hormones because the skin all over his body was too severely inflamed to treat without corticosteroids. His IgE RIST (radioimmunosorbent test) values were 335,000 IU/ml, and his IgE RAST (radioallergosorbent test) values in response to a house-dust antigen, a house tick antigen and a cat skin crumb antigen showed more than 100 units (measurable upper limit: 100 units). Additionally, his serum cortisol was 1.2 g/dl, which was a level too low to protect him.

After this treatment, his skin inflammation appeared to disappear, although his IgE RIST and IgE RAST values did not decrease. Naturally, his skin was red from several months of the allergic reaction inflammation. He again began to suffer from severe itching. Finally, he suffered from bacterial infections on his skin from having scratched himself with dirty fingernails; thus, bacteria were present continuously.

Treatments that he received at other hospitals were nearly identical to those at the first hospital. As a result, he had repeated recurrences of the dermatitis.

His mother brought him to the authors' clinic to receive psychosomatic treatments.

The Plan of Treatment

Vaseline containing red pepper to cool down his itching and antibiotics to sterilize bacteria on his skin were prescribed.

At first, free play therapy was provided once a week by his psychologist, followed by friendly, psychoanalytical play therapy and Daseinsanalysis (including sand play therapy).

Continuous counseling and psychotherapy were provided for his mother because his mother appeared very suppressive and irritable toward him.

For several weeks, a 0.5 mg dose of Lorazepam was prescribed nightly when he could not sleep because of severe itching over his entire body.

The Course of PNIP Treatment

1. Stage One

    At first, although the therapist attempted to play with him freely, he played by himself, ignoring the therapist. After several sessions, he gradually began playing with the therapist.

2. Stage Two

    He regressed to acting like a baby for several sessions. He gradually began to treat his disease with detachment after his psychologist began sand play therapy.

3. Stage Two to Three

    He treated his disease with complete detachment, accompanied by displays of explosive emotion. He began to fight against his atopic dermatitis directly with the therapist. The theme of his Sand Play was "war." He began sharing his life history through telling stories.

4. Stage Four

    During his fight against his dermatitis, he sometimes became violent and/or cried. Sand Play gradually revealed his unconscious past life until about three years old.

5. Stage Five

    In this way, his disease left him after approximately 6 years.

The Results of His Chemical Tests

His dermatitis, including inflammation, gradually began to improve approximately one year after the first visit. His IgE RIST values decreased to 32,050 IU/ml, and his IgE RAST values decreased to less than 100 units. His serum cortisol level was 3.6 g/dl.

The same treatments were continued for approximately 5 years. At that time, his skin appeared normal except for a few spots. His IgE RIST values were 826 IU/ml, and his IgE RAST values were 45 units, which are still higher than normal levels. His serum cortisol levels increased to 6.8 g/dl.

The treatment based on psychoneuroimmunopathological techniques will be continued until his dermatitis is completely improved and he shows reduced IgE RIST and IgE RAST values. **(Figure below)**

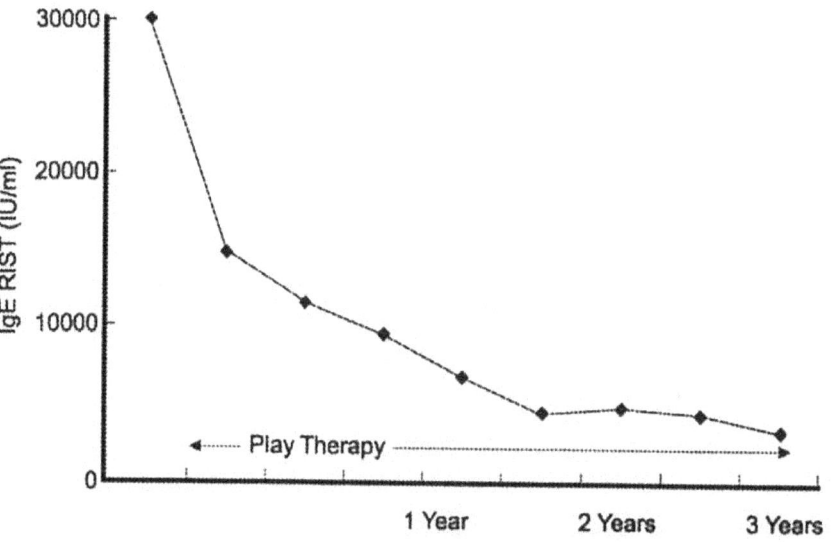

Figure: The variations of IgE RIST levels on this case.

Discussion

The author introduced seven cases who were suffering from severely disturbing allergic diseases and presented a typical course of treatment using PNIP. The psychoneuroimmunopathological (PNIP) approach and the characteristics of these cases are as follows:

These cases showed improvement without any anti-allergic agents, although they were brought in for treatment for allergic reactions.

These cases showed severely high IgE RIST and IgE RAST values, which were decreased to lower levels, corresponding to improvement in the disease.

These cases showed low levels of serum cortisol, which increased to higher levels, corresponding to improvement in the disease.

Daseinsanalysis in play therapy was very effective as a cathartic technique for improvement.

The counseling and psychotherapy for the mother were effective in the patient's improvement because she gradually accepted him more naturally.

In this case, corticosteroid hormones were not given, although today it is common sense to prescribe corticosteroid hormones for severe allergic diseases including atopic dermatitis, whether as ointments or oral drugs. Therefore, contemporary and traditional treatments for allergic diseases were denied by these authors' treatment.

As a result, because it was suspected that IgE is controlled by the brain, it will be most important to analyze and create an opportunity for catharsis to lower severely high IgE values.

Allergic diseases usually appear during the period of rebelliousness, particularly the first period of rebelliousness. Children in the period of rebelliousness are often so nervous, weak and sensitive to changes in circumstance that they are susceptible to illnesses from emotional and/or somatic factors, which are further causes of such illnesses. Certain psychopathological approaches work to elevate defense mechanisms such as immunological and hormonal abilities.

However, even today, psychopathological treatments are not always provided for such children. Staff who provide treatment for children, particularly in the rebellious period, should provide these psychopathological treatments.

When such psychopathological treatments are provided, fewer drugs with side effects will need to be prescribed.

These treatment methods for allergic diseases should become the basic approach.

Furthermore, children suffering from allergic diseases may have a constitutional vulnerability to allergic reactions, but often they have psychological problems from birth. For example, they might be born into families where they are not really welcome; consequently, their positive emotions and thoughts may continuously be suppressed, and/or they may have received implicit or explicit ill treatment. Children in such situations suffer from allergic diseases during the first period of rebelliousness because they never show their emotions positively. Thus, emotional disturbance might appear as somatoform allergic disorders because children have allergic constitutions, which makes them easily susceptible to allergic diseases. Furthermore, children have only a few means to express their wronged and suppressed minds.

It is commonly believed in the medical world, particularly in allergology, that there is little relationship between emotion and allergic response; thus, the primary forms of treatment for allergic diseases are medications instead of psychological treatment.

Unfortunately, it is difficult to treat children with only medication because of severe side effects that might be lethal in children but not in adults.

Therefore, the "Experimental Study 1" mentioned above is still not accepted in the medical world.

Fortunately, the results of using PNIP show the relationship between allergic responses and emotion, including the mind and spirit.

Thus, PNIP is revealed to be the most useful and effective treatment, but it is difficult to learn and understand PNIP. In fact, the PNIP procedures through play therapy were undergoing development as they were performed. You can see here that the patient's IgE RIST levels dropped from 335,000 to 826 IU/ml.

Conclusion

These cases led the authors to conclude that PNIP will be the safest and most effective treatment method for severe allergic diseases abandoned by specialists.

References:

Nash, M. R.: Salient findings in hypnosis literature: Int J Clin Exp Hyp. 50:202, 2002.

Cowings, R. S., Toscano, W. B.: Autogenic-feedback training exercise superior to promethazine for control of motion sickness symptoms. J Clin Pharmcol 40:1154, 2000.

Lekmander, M.: The immne systemis affected by psychological factors. High stress levels can change susceptibility to infection and allergy. Review. Swedish. PMID: 10584543

Wyler-Harper, J., et al.: Hypnosis and allergic response. Sweiz Med. Wochenschr Suppl 62:67, 1994.

Staudenmayer, H., Selner, J. C.: Neuropsychophysiology during relaxation in generalized, universal 'allergic' reactivity to the environment: a comparison study. J Psychosom Res 34:259, 1990.

Collison, D. R.: Which asthmatic patients should be treated by hypnotherapy? Med J Augst. 1:776, 1975.

O'Neill, D., Malcomson, K.: Results of treatment of chronic vasomotor rhinitis. II. Response to psychological treatment. Br Med J 1:554, 1954.

Nielsen, R. G., Husby, S.: Eosinophilic oesophagitis: epidemiology, clinical aspects, and association to allergy. J Pediatr Gastroenterol Nutr. 45:281, 2007.

Hodges, M. G., Keane-Myers, A. M.: Classification of ocular allergy. Curr Opin Allergy Clin Immunol. 7:429, 2007.

Larche, M.: Regulatory T cells in allergy and asthma. Chest. 132:1007, 2007.

Butterfield, J. H.: Treatment of hypereosinophilic syndromes with predonisone, hydroxyure and interfection. Immunol Allergy Clin North Am. 27:493, 2007.

Rachelefsky, G. F.: Difficult-to-control asthma: underlying factors, clinical implications, and treatment strategies. Curr Med Res Opin., 2007

Tofte, S.: Atopic dermatitis. Nurs Cin North Am. 42:407, 2007.

Tetu, L., Didier, A: Allergic disease treatments classic and innovative therapeutics. Rev Prat. 57:1339, 2007.

Busse, W. W., et al.: Effect of omalizumab on the need for rescue systemic corticosteroid treatment in patients with moderate-to-severe persistent IgE-mediated allergic asthma: a pooled analysis. Curr Med Res Opin., 2007.

Reidulf, G. Watten, Asbjorn, O., Faleide: Behavioral and normal health profile in childhood hay fever. British J Health Psychology, 1: 349, 1996.

Asbjorn, O. Fleide, Vigdis, K. J., Sissel, U., Reidulf, G. W.: Children at risk of allergic development: The parents' Dyadic Relationship. Psychother Psychosom. 49:223, 1988.

HAJIME JOZUKA, M.D.

Practical Applications of PNIP in Treating Chronic Fatigue Syndrome

Introduction

The pathogenesis of Chronic Fatigue Syndrome (CSF) has never been clarified, although clinical symptoms, including immune responses, have been classified as a syndrome for a long time.

Many studies, particularly about immune responses, have been performed over the years. Many reports described the reduction of natural killer cell activity in their studies because CSF clients easily contract viral-infections. However, only a few studies examining the relationship between endocrine responses and CSF are available. Furthermore, no psychoneuroendocrinoimmunological study has been available, as far as the authors know.

Given this state of affairs, treatments for a client suffering from chronic fatigue syndrome were conducted using Daseinsanalysis and psychoneuroimmunopathology (PNIP). As a result, the client completely recovered from CSF, and for more than five years no symptoms have been observed in the client.

In this study, a CFS client treated by PNIP will be discussed.

Subjects

1) PINP treatments were provided for five clients suffering from CFS. All of their profiles and results including age, sex, symptoms, clinical findings, treatment methods, and intervals until remission are presented in the following table.

Table: Chronic Fatigue Syndrome treated using PNIP

Age	Sex	Symptoms	Treatment	Interval until Remission	Findings
39	M	General Muscle Rigidity	AT, Counseling	8 years	NK cell act. 2.5 %Fluvoxamine+MilnacipraneCPK: 3500 U/LDiazepam intravenous inject.
41	M	general fatigue, muscle pain	AT, Counseling	7 years	Slight fever, NK cell act. 6.2 % FluvoxamineCPK: 3020 U/L Diazepam intravenous inject.
42	M	general muscle rigidity, Gait disturbance, unknown infection	Meditation, Counseling	8 years+	Diazepam and antibiotics; NK cell act. 9.5 %, CPK: 2500 U/L inject., Paroxetine
46	M	general fatigue, partial muscle rigidity	AT, Counseling	7 years	NK cell act. 4.8 %, CPK: 952 U/L Fluvoxamine, Diazepam inject.
48	M	general muscle pain, gait disturbance	Short counseling, Paroxetine	3 years	Diazepam inject. NK cell act. 17 %, CPK: 450 U/L

AT: autogenic training; inject: intravenous injection; act.: activity; CPK: creatinine phosphokinesis

All of the patients had already been misdiagnosed as having severe depression, immune deficiency syndrome, or hyper-creatinine phosphokinese-emia, but they had never received treatment at top rated medical schools.

A Typical Case Suffering From CFS
Case
A 41-year-old male holding a managerial position in a big company.

Personality: Type A behavior pattern (Type A scores by Jenkins Activity Survey: 98 %, Intelligent Quality: 170 %).

Chief complaints: general fatigue, easy fatigability, general muscle pain and rigidity, reduction of activity, sleep rhythm disturbances, slight fever and vulnerability to viral infections.

Some Bio-chemical Findings
- Serum CPK: 3020 U/L
- SScrum Myoglobine: 120 ng/ml
- SNatural killer cell activity: 6.2 %
- SInterleukin-2 productivity: 560 IU/ml,
- SDehydroepiandrosterone: 1.2 ng/ml
- SSerum cortisol: 2.4 g/dl

Treatment
- SAutogenic training, counseling and Daseinsanalysis
- SFluvoxamine 50 100 mg/day + Diazepam 15 mg/day
- SDHEA 200 mg/day
- SDiazepam (intravenous injection) 10 mg/day

Course of Illness
The client joined the company as an executive trainee. He never noticed or felt overworked, although he usually worked more than 15 hours a day. About twice a week, he worked overnight. Although this lifestyle continued until his late thirties, he jogged approximately 20 km every day.

He began to notice general muscle pain when he was running. In addition, it began to be difficult to get up in the morning due to general fatigue and general muscle pain. Moreover, he could not get enough sleep.

At last, he visited a hospital and received treatment. Although he had been treated for severe depression for more than one year, he did not improve; thus, he visited the authors' clinic. He was diagnosed as a typical case of chronic fatigue syndrome.

Course of Treatment

The treatment plan prescribed for his chronic fatigue syndrome was as follows:

Suggestions for his daily regimen: rest, relaxation, and some stretching. The purpose was to alter his Type A behavior pattern lifestyle by relaxation of the muscles accompanied by Daseinsanalysis; because his personality was so rigid and abnormal, Daseinsanalysis was prescribed to clarify his pathogeneses.

Autogenic training was performed at the clinic once a week, and music therapy was performed before and after autogenic training for an hour. The purpose was to provide a period of relaxation time in his life.

Prescription of SSRI (Fluvoxamine: 50 mg/2/day for 3 months and then 100 mg/2/day). The purpose of this prescription was to elevate his natural killer cell activity, dehydroepiandrosterone, and cortisol values.

Diazepam 10 mg venous injections every second day. The purpose of the injections was to relax his muscles.

Prescription of DHEA 50 mg/2/day. The purpose of this prescription was to elevate his immune responses and repair and recovery abilities.

Treatment began with the staff at the clinic according to the above plan. In the beginning, it was difficult to treat him because his personality and his Type A behavior pattern were not easily changeable. He could not forget his work. Thus, his pathological symptoms were not easily changeable until these fundamental characteristics improved. Because his personality and behavior pattern included rigidity, he received treatment so regularly that he acquired relaxation techniques more rapidly than any other client. Diazepam injections were effective for muscle relaxation, and as a result, there was no need to increase the dosage.

He received treatment and worked every day; consequently, he repeatedly swung between improvement and relapses. His boss finally ordered him to rest until he was fully recovered. He decided to take a rest and returned to receive treatment including relaxation.

From then on, his symptoms gradually decreased, and he seldom suffered from viral infections. With this improvement, his natural killer cell activity increased to 32 %.

Seven years after the first visit, all of his symptoms had completely subsided, but he continues to take medicine because he is worried that he will suffer a recurrence.

He returned to work but was unable to work as hard as he had in the past. Although he does not work as hard, he is more highly valued than in the past.

Discussion and Conclusion

The authors attempted to treat five patients suffering from chronic fatigue syndrome; the details of a typical case are described in this study. At first, chronic fatigue syndrome showed findings similar to severe depression, i.e., a reduction of natural killer cell activity, DHEA and serum cortisol levels. Symptoms of chronic fatigue syndrome are very similar to severe depression, with the addition of general muscle pain.

These observations led us to speculate that the pathogeneses for chronic fatigue syndrome and severe depression might be the same because the courses of the two illnesses are so similar to one another.

Although chronic fatigue syndrome appears similar to severe depression, the disorders are essentially different psychopathological diseases. In terms of pathogenesis, they differ from one another. The point where they coincide is the immune response. As a result, treatment for chronic fatigue syndrome will differ from the treatment for severe depression. In addition, although clients who suffered from severe depression did rest, the client who suffered from chronic fatigue syndrome never kept his promise when the therapist ordered him to take a long rest. The fundamental life values of a person who suffers from CFS differ from those of a severely depressed person, including their definitions of words.

When the therapist suggested that he rest his mind and body for a month, the CFS patient might not only not yield to the suggestion but might also begin some training to improve his body, compared to a person with severe depression who would be more likely to accept the suggestion.

This typical case clearly displays that it is important to treat chronic fatigue syndrome based on the philosophy of PNIP.

Conclusion of Practical Clinical Aspects

Although only five typical cases were presented in this study, all of the cases were treated with Daseinsanalysis based on the philosophy of PNIP. In each of these cases, the PNIP methods of treatment were actually the proper methods to have been be used.

It is most important to evaluate the client's degree of stress according to the Stress Theory. After the stage is explained to the client, superficial treatment to care for symptoms and basic treatments to alleviate fundamental psycho-pathogeneses should be performed.

The actual methods of psychoneuroimmunopathology can be explained as follows:

Daseinsanalysis (psychopathological approaches), whether concrete or abstract, should be performed for all clients because entire diseases, disorders, and unhealthy situations advance based on psychogeneses. When these approaches have been explained completely, neuro-endocrino-immunological abilities will increase and be elevated in all clients.

Of course, these psychological approaches include laughter training, relaxation training, and other behavioral training because they are otherwise ineffective.

SSRIs, SNRI and dehydroepiandrosterone are important additional treatments that should be prescribed according to the individual client's needs.

Psychoneuroimmunopathological approaches are the simplest method of treatment; thus, many clients will be able to receive them.

However, these methods will be more effective for clients only when the entire staff provides them patiently and discreetly.

References

Baker, R., Shaw, E.: Diagnosis and management of chronic fatigue syndrome or myalgic encephalomyelitis (or encephalopathy): summary of NICE guidance. BMJ.335:446,2007.

Guo, J.: Chronic fatigue syndrome treated by acupuncture and moxibustion in combination with psychological approaches in 310 cases. J Tradit Clin Med.27:92, 2007.

Brown, R. J.: Introduction to the special issue on medically unexpected symptoms: Background and future directions. Clin Psyhcol Rev. 27:769, 2007.

Jansen, N. W., et al.: Aetiology of prolonged fatigue among workers. An overview of findings from the Maastricht Cohort Study. Tijdsch Psychiatr. 49:537, 2007.

Carville, S.F., et al.: EULAR evidence based recommendations for the management of fibromyalgia syndrome. Ann Rheum Dis. 2007.

Perrin, R. N.: Lymphatic drainage of the neuraxis in chronic fatigue syndrome: a hyperthetical model for the cranial rhythmic impulse. J Am Osteopath Assoc. 107:218, 2007.

Masuda, A., Menemoto, T., Tei, C.: A new treatment: thermal therapy forchronic fatigue syndrome. Nippon Rinhso. 65:1093, 2007.

Murakami, M.: Consideration for treatment of chronic fatigue syndrome. 65:1089, 2007.

Wyller, B., et al.: Treatment of chronic fatigue and other orthostatic intolerance with propranolol. J Pedatr. 150:654, 2007.

Knoop, H., et al.: Is cognitive behaviour therapy for chronic fatigue syndrome also effective for pain syndromes? BehavRes Ther. 45:2034, 2007.

Wyller, V. B.: The chronic fatigue syndrome—an update. Acta-Neurolo Scand Suppl. 187:7, 2007.

Young, J. L., Redmond, J. C.: Fibromyalgia, chronic fatigue, and adult attention deficit hyperactivity disorder in the adult: a case study. Psychopharmacol Bull. 40:118, 2007.

Wearden, A. G., Chew-Graham, C.: Managing chronic fatigue syndrome in U.K. primary care: challenges and opportunities. Chonic Illn. 2:143, 2006.

Practical Application in Coronary Heart Disease—"Prevention and Treatment of Coronary Heart Disease Using PNIP"

Introduction

It was not clear whether serotonin selective reuptake inhibitors (SSRIs) were effective for coronary heart disease from the studies about SSRIs. Many reports claim that many SSRIs are harmful and/or cause coronary heart disease, particularly cardiovascular infarction. Other studies maintain that some SSRIs prevent and effectively treat myocardial infarction and other coronary heart diseases (CHDs). Recently, the latter studies and reports are increasing, despite other studies maintaining that tricyclic agents are harmful to myocardial infarction.

Therefore, the authors would like to describe the effects of SSRIs on coronary heart diseases by reviewing several cases.

Subjects and Methods

Subjects

Five clients suffering from CHD came to receive treatment for the following psychiatric complaints: depressive mood, anxiety, and activity reduction, which interfered with their usual lifestyle. All of the patients were in such serious condition that they had no option other than to visit the authors to receive PNIP treatments. They had been told by specialists in the best university hospitals, "Your disease will never be controllable or curable in the department of circulatory organs because your disease is caused by autonomic nerve unbalance. We can take no responsibility for your disease. You must be treated by the departments of Psychiatry or Psychosomatic Medicine."

The initial motivations of the clients when they came to us are shown in **Table 1**.

Methods

Treatment using PNIP was provided for each client as shown in **Table 2**.

At first, each client was prescribed an SSRI, antianxietic agents, and other medications.

Daseinsanalysis, sand play therapy, and alcohol abstinence therapy were provided for the clients depending on their needs.

Results

The results for all of the clients are shown in **Table 3**.

All of the clients lived at least ten years after their first visit, but clients No. 1 and 2 were admitted to the cardiac care unit of a hospital as a result of frequent attacks after ceasing to take SSRIs at their own discretion for several weeks. No. 5 was admitted because of suffering from ascites due to liver cirrhosis.

None of the clients have experienced any symptoms other than some accidents for more than ten years.

Table 1: Profiles of the Coronary Heart Disease Clients

#	Sex	Age	Diagnosis and Main Symptoms at the Departments of Circulatory Organs
1	M	38	frequent attacks of vasospastic angina from the use of usual medications
2	M	43	frequent attacks of vasospastic angina from the use of usual medications
3	M	48	frequent attacks of angina pectoris due to/from hard work (Type A behavior pattern)
4	M	58	uncontrollable attacks of angina pectoris and hypertension
5	M	62	myocardial infarction after an operation and alcohol dependence

Table 2. Treatments

Client#	Added Medications	Psychotherapeutic Approaches
1	Fluvoxamine 50 mg/day	Daseinsanalysis and Autogenic Training
2	Fluvoxamine 50 mg/day	Sand Play Therapy and Autogenic Training
3	Paroxetine 10 mg/day Flutoprazepam 2 mg/day	Daseinsanalysis and Autogenic Training
4	Paroxetine 20 mg/day	Daseinsanalysis and Autogenic Training
5	Fluvoxamine 100 mg/day Flutoprazepam 2 mg/day Glycyrrhizinic acid 100 ml/day	Alcohol Abstinence Therapy and Sand Play Therapy

Table 3. Results

Client No	Main symptoms	Asymptomatic Period	Situation
1	Subsided	eight years	working
2	Subsided	seven years	working
3	Subsided	more than ten years	working
4	Improved	more than ten years	working
5	No Attack	more than ten years	working

Discussion

The author described five clients suffering from coronary heart disease whose disease was severe and uncontrollable by circulatory organ specialists. All of the clients returned to a controllable condition using PNIP. All of them likely would have died from their previous attack if they had not been ordered to enroll in a department of psychosomatic medicine or psychiatry.

The medical etiology of the disease in Cases No. 1 and 2 is still unknown, but their symptoms, including pathological mechanisms, are similar to one another.

Cases No. 1 and No. 2 each suffered only one attack after the first month of PNIP treatment. Cases No. 3, 4, and 5 had no attacks for more than ten years after visiting the author or beginning PNIP treatment.

The author knows that in the past SSRIs were considered a risk factor for myocardial infarction. Recently, because of progress in psychosomatic and psychopharmacological medicine, it is increasingly being demonstrated that the mechanism of serotonin selective reuptake inhibition is effective in preventing the appearance and the relapse of attacks in coronary heart disease.

The author's treatment (PNIP) is classified as a psychoanalytic and pharmacologic treatment. Of course, all of the clients experienced stage 1 to stage 5. Unfortunately, clients who suffered from CHD had many psychosomatic risk factors in their lifestyles and life histories, and they had to take time to address many aspects other than their disease. Had they devoted energy to their treatment even longer, they might still be living without anxiety or fear of relapse.

It does not need to be said that these five clients who suffered from severe coronary heart and myocardial diseases fought against their diseases and won.

Conclusion

It was clarified that PNIP is a very effective means to control and prevent coronary heart disease and myocardial diseases.

As a result, physicians should prescribe SSRIs and Daseinsanalysis when they diagnose a client with coronary heart disease and/or myocardial diseases.

Appendix

The author will describe nine exceptional cases. (The profile of the clients at their first visit is shown in Table 4). These cases have been treated for depression or other psychosomatic diseases and received Daseinsanalytic counseling to cure or prevent disease by taking SSRIs or SNRI for more than ten years. Because they had been diagnosed with brain arterial aneurysms, they lived in constant fear that the aneurysm would burst.

Unfortunately, all of the clients suffered brain arterial bleeding within six to seven years after visiting the author. Although they were admitted to the hospital because they were suffering from sudden severe headache, all of them were discharged within several days after taking hemostatic agents. Furthermore, thorough examinations showed only small bleeding lesions. They are still healthy today.

It might be difficult to explain why they are healthy, but some small effect might result from the use of PNIP and Daseinsanalysis including SSRIs. Because some reports researching the relationship between cerebral arteries, depression and SSRIs are available, the mechanisms of prevention and treatment using SSRIs and some psychotherapy will be described within a short time.

Although the author confirmed the presence of a brain arterial aneurysm by angiographs of brain arteries, the author could not clarify the mechanism of improvement of an aneurysm. These nine cases have no aneurysms today; nevertheless, the author confirmed the existence of brain arterial aneurysms at the first visit.

The author hopes to show the mechanism of the improvement of brain arterial aneurysms as soon as possible.

Table 4. Clients Suffering from a Brain Arterial Aneurysm at Their First Visit.

Client	Main Symptom	Aneurysm	Medication	Prognosis
38 M	Irritable bowel syndrome	8 mm x 3	Fluvoxamine	No Sequela
40 M	Severe depression	10 mm	Fluvoxamine	No Sequela
44 M	Severe depression	12 mm	Paroxetine	No Sequela
44 F	Ulcerative colitis	8 mm x 5	Paroxetine	No Sequela
45 F	Irritable bowel syndrome	9 mm	Fluvoxamine	No Sequela
47 M	Severe depression	5-9 mm x 3	Milnacipran	No Sequela
50 F	Panic disorder	8-9 mm x 2	Paroxetine	No Sequela
52 F	Severe depression	9 mm	Milnacipran	No Sequela
53 M	Severe depression	5-9 mm x 2	Milnacipran	No Sequela

M: male, F: female Because all of the clients were afraid of relapse, they continued taking medicine.

References:

Xiong, G. L., et al.: Prognosis of patients taking selective serotonin reuptake inhibitors before coronary artery bypass grafting. Am J Cardiol. 98:42-7, 2006.

Sauer, W. H., Berlin, J. A., Kimmel, S. E.: Effect of antidepressant and their relative affinity for the serotonin transporter on the risk of myocardial infarction. Circulation. 108:32-6, 2003.

Rose, S. P., Miyazaki, M.: Pharmacologic treatment of depression in patients with heart disease. Psychosom Med. 67: S54-7, 2005.

Schlienger, R. G., Meier, C. R.: Effect of selective serotonin reuptake inhibitors on platelet activation: can they prevent acute myocardial infarction? Am J Cardiovasc Drugs. 3:149-62, 2003.

Berkman, L. F., et al.: Effects of depression and low perceived social support on clinical events after myocardial infarction: the Enhancing Recovery in Coronary Heart Disease Patients (ENRICHD) Randomized Trial. JAMA. 289, 3106-16, 2003.

Sauer, W. H., Berlin, J. A., Kimmel, S. E.: Selective serotonin reuptake inhibitors and myocardial infarction. Circulation. 104:1894-8, 2001.

Meier, C. R., Schlinger, J. A., Jick, H.: Use of selective serotonin reuptake inhibitors and risk of developing firm time acute myocardial infarction. Br. J Clin Pharmcol. 52:179-84, 2001.

Strik, J. J., et al.: Cardiac side-effects of two selective serotonin reuptake inhibitors in middle-aged and elderly depressed patients. Int Cliin Psychophrmacol. 13:263-7, 1999.

Singhal, A. B., et al.: SSRI and statin use increase the risk for vasospasm after subarachnoid hemorrhage. Neurology. 2005. 64:1008-3.

Nobler, M. S., Mann, J. J., Sackeim, H. A.: Serotonin, cerebral blood flow, and cerebral metabolic rate in geriatric severe depression and normal aging. Brain Res Brain Rev 1999, 30,

250-63: Review.
Fricchiene, G. L., Woznicki, R. M., Klesmser, J., Vlay, S. E.: Vasoconstrictive effect and SSRIs. J Clin Psychiatry 1993, 54:71-2.

PNIP Based on Psychopathology

PNIP based on psychopathology was established not only for the sake of research but also for use as a practical therapeutic method.

The authors provide a summary of the practical psychotherapy methods and of immune ability responses as follows:

1. Stage 1 occurs when the therapist and the client become acquainted.
2. Stages 2 and 3 – The client defines his own disease and identifies it as an enemy while gradually developing resistance to it. In these stages, the therapist is regarded as the leader. When the client feels that he/she is fully accepted, the relief causes the client's immune responses to lower. To deepen the relationship between the therapist and the client, the client begins to tell his/her life story and to describe his/her lifestyle until the onset of the disease, thus digging deeper and wider.
3. As the therapy progresses, the client's immune ability gradually improves. Daseinsanalysis had previously begun with the client's regard for the process.
4. Stage 4 – The enemy is observed as completely separate from the client when the client begins to relate to the therapist, who is now regarded as a comrade. At that time, the immune ability is at its highest levels until the enemy is destroyed.
5. Stage 5 – This is the triumphant moment, the remission stage.

This method is defined as psychoneuroimmunopathology based on Daseinsanalysis. (**Figure**) In other words, psychoneuroimmunopathology includes Daseinsanalysis. The clients' phenomenological descriptions of their life history and lifestyle are the most important methods in Daseinsanalysis and psychoneuroimmunopathology.

Thus, psychoneuroimmunopathology includes Daseinsanalysis, and Daseinsanalysis includes psychoneuroimmunopathology. The practical methodology will be derived from the theory.

Psychoneuroimmunopathology is the easiest theoretical and practical method used to treat "incurable" clients.

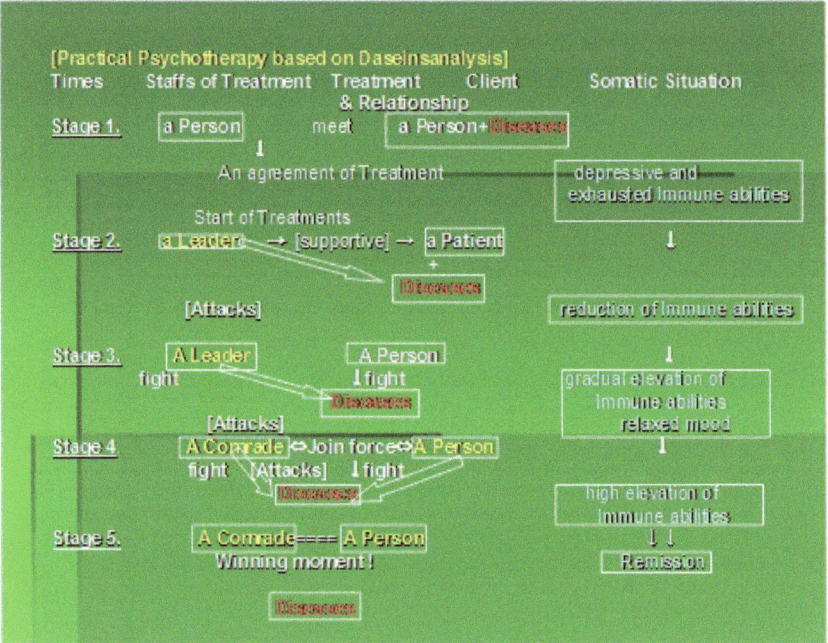

Figure: Practical Psychotherapy Based on Daseinsanalysis

Fundamental Philosophy of Psychoneuroimmunopathology Medical Anthropological Psychopathology

Discussion of the Fundamental Philosophy of PNIP Medical Anthropological Psychopathology

The authors will discuss the fundamental philosophy of PNIP, which is a simple method based on a wide variety philosophical principles. There are many people who suffer from incurable diseases in the world, and the author feels they can be helped by receiving this easy treatment, which any physician can master. PNIP including Daseinsanalysis is exactly the treatment they need. It may be easy for physicians to treat tonsillitis using only antibiotics, but people think that it is extremely difficult to treat a client who was informed by a specialist that the time of his/her death from an incurable disease is approaching.

Fortunately, the author discovered this easy method to treat clients suffering from such "incurable" diseases. Any physician can easily use this method after having served an apprenticeship. No specialist is required to exert extreme intellectual effort to master the method, compared to liaison psychiatry and psychosomatic medicine.

Once the method is mastered, one need not fear any incurable disease.

Pathogenesis— Fundamental Recognition of an Unhealthy Human Being (Figure 1)

We all know that the frontal lobes of the brain facilitate the peripheral circumstances. We could even say that it is responsible for creating the human relationships that our society is founded upon. This brain function can also make a human being generally unhealthy. When this unhealthiness develops, a human being suffers from diseases. Furthermore, because schizophrenia and manic illness might be a result of reduced dopamine, human beings suffering from these conditions might not be aware of their situation.

Therefore, the highest brain functions might make a human being unhealthy.

Existence of Human Beings (Figure 2)

As we move through our daily lives, we generate our own existence, we encounter many types of problems, and we become stressed and exhausted.

Stress makes us prone to some diseases, and when some people suffer from some diseases, they become depressed; the depressive state weakens their immune systems, which makes the disease severe. This eventually becomes a vicious cycle.

PNIP can break the vicious cycle by combining antidepressants with psychotherapy. PNIP suddenly reverses the trend of decreasing immune abilities by increasing those immune abilities. Increased immune abilities eventually lead to general recovery or at least to remission.

Because human beings are constantly worrying about their circumstances and always have problems in their life history and lifestyles, they will often be exhausted. When individuals suffer from disease, sometimes as a result of stress, they become depressed. It is well known that depression causes reduced immune function.

When such phenomena occur, some people will succumb to serious disease. The vicious cycle starts in the human being.

The fundamental philosophy of PNIP treatments is to disrupt this vicious cycle.

First, the depression must be treated. It is easy to treat depression superficially by providing antidepressants and supportive psychotherapy. However, when the diseases are severe and difficult to treat, special complicated treatments, mentioned above, are required.

Initially, SSRIs, including SNRIs, should be prescribed as agents to elevate NK activity, and DHEA should be prescribed as a neurosteroid hormone repair and recovery agent. Special medicines, for example, Glycyrrhizinic acid for hepato-cellular destruction, anti-allergic agents for allergic diseases and Diazepam for CFS, should be prescribed depending on the prevalent symptoms of disease.

It is a deeply interesting phenomenon that the number of clients suffering from malignant neoplasms has been decreasing for the past ten years in correlation with the increasing mass production of SSRIs. (Figure 2)

The "Seesaw" Phenomenon

Let us discuss human defense mechanisms a bit further. From an immunological viewpoint, human defense mechanisms are not so simple because if they were, everyone would have noticed the relationship between the T cell line and natural killer cell responses. In other words, although the T cell line responds against bacteria, with which the person has had contact prior, the T cell line does not respond against viruses and neoplasms, with which they have never had prior contact.

On the one hand, when a sudden invader or acute stressor that the T cell line has never encountered before enters a human being, the T cell line cannot function as a defense mechanism. Only natural killer cells are activated. Most likely the frontal lobe of the brain activates the natural killer cell defense mechanism.

On the other hand, when invaders or stressors that the T-cell line has had prior contact with enter the body, such as familiar bacteria, the T-cell line immediately responds against them, instead of the natural killer cells.

Thus, the responsibilities of the defense mechanisms differ from one another. Usually, the T cell line is responsible against chronic stressors and/or invaders including bacteria, and natural killer cells respond against acute stressors including viruses.

These reactions are defined as the "Seesaw" phenomenon. In other words, when T cells are elevated as a defense, natural killer cells are never elevated. When natural killer cells are activated, the T cell line never moves.

This balance system is likely controlled by the frontal lobe of the brain. In addition, it is thought that all defense mechanisms might be controlled by levels of -endorphins and enkephalin in the frontal lobe of the brain. Thus, it is suspected that there is a deep relationship between thought and defense mechanisms in the frontal lobe of the brain.

On the one hand, relaxation such autogenic training, laughter therapy, aroma therapy and music therapy (and sexual intercourse) elevate natural killer cell activity to guard against sudden stressors. On the other hand, sudden stress elevates natural killer cell activity. These opposite phenomena might be a result of the elevation of -endorphin. Furthermore, T cell lines do not move in such situations; the T-cell line works only in stable or depressive states in human beings. Thus, by the differing responsibilities of their immunological systems, human beings should be guarded against stressors and invaders and thereby be able to recover from diseases.

Unfortunately, it is common that when the T cell line increases, natural killer cell activity decreases, and when natural killer cell activity increases, T cell line activity decreases. Maintaining this balance might be difficult, particularly in humans ("Seesaw phenomenon between T cell and NK cell": discovered by the author).

It is difficult to strike a balance between the different immunological theories, particularly the "Cosmic Phenomenology" by Heidegger. Usually, because of former cell elevation, a bacterial infection leaves the client, but the client then begins to suffer from a viral infection and/or neoplasm. The same situation might occur when natural killer cell activity increases and when the client recovers from a viral infection and/or neoplasm.

Only PNIP will be able to create a balance between activation of the T cell line and natural killer cell activity.

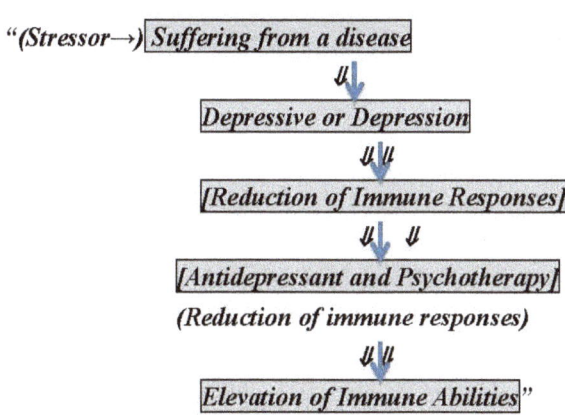

Antidepressant: SSRIs or SNRI+DHEA   psychotherapy: Daseinsanalysis

Figure 2: Existence of a Human Being

Fundamental Theory of Existential Philosophy in Psychosomatics (Figure 3)

Today, it is a known and interesting fact that superficial psychotherapy and cognitive behavioral therapy are never as effective against terminal diseases as traditional psychoanalysis.

Let us consider the difference between contemporary treatments and traditional German psychotherapy. The latter analyzes, and the former was never close to such an achievement.

Kimura described the existence of human beings in the spatiotemporal order, which is defined as "ante festum" (before), "intra festum" (during), and "post festum" (after). These three classifications relate to the phenomenological onset of an attack. Therefore, depression (including diseases caused by another disease) exists "post festum." An attack (including diseases that include an attack) exists in "intra festum." Diseases manifesting as anxiety about the future exist in "ante festum." Entire existences are defined based on phenomenology. It is rare to find neoplasms in clients suffering from schizophrenia, which is an "ante festum" disease, because it is impossible for that person to conceptualize anything that does not exist at present. The present immediately becomes the past. Therefore, the therapist and client analyze the continuity of existence in Daseinsanalysis. As a result, they both look forward by analyzing and extrapolating from the recent past into the present, including not only life events but also time itself.

Diseases classified as existing "intra festum" include epilepsy, schizoaffective disorders, coronary heart attack, and pain-attacks in the gall bladder or pancreas, etc. The only disease classified as "ante festum" might be schizophrenia. Many diseases are classified as existing "post festum," such as all diseases that involve depression, for example, neoplasms, autoimmune diseases including rheumatoid arthritis, congenital diseases, etc.

Martin Heidegger and Medard Boss further promulgated this concept, as mentioned before. Heidegger stressed the importance of insight; Boss explained psychosomatic medicine based on existential philosophy, and Kimura explained the idea of spatiotemporal existence.

Heidegger considered that an individual understands existence only when he understands and accepts death. Heidegger therefore thought that only human beings are able to have insight into spatiotemporal theory.

Medard Boss combined the depth psychology of Freud with the existential philosophy of Heidegger and established Daseinsanalysis based on phenomenology. Daseinsanalysis (existential psychology) combined human psychology with Heidegger's phenomenological view of human existence. The broad interpretation of Daseinsanalysis attempts to reconcile the dualities of human existence through a criticism of natural scientific psychology and psychiatry. Daseinsanalysis was established by Ludwig Binswanger and was spread by Medard Boss, who was devoted to Heidegger. His Daseinsanalysis fundamentally differs from the "psychoanalyse existentiele" of Jean Paul Sartre and the "Existenzanalyse" of Viktor Frankl.

Dasein is defined as a being's awareness of being in the world. Medard Boss founded the Swiss Society for Daseinsanalysis in 1970 and the Zurich Institute for Daseinsanalytic Psychotherapy and Psychosomatics in 1971, later known as the Medard Boss Foundation. Based on their studies, the idea that the therapist and the client fight together against the disease is called Daseinsanalysis. Observing the disease from a common perspective and fighting against it with a combined effort is significantly better than just being dependent on SSRIs.

Daseinsanalysis as put forward by Heidegger, Boss and Kimura maintains that the concept of spirit and mind differs from brain phenomena. Moreover, their argument is that mind is body and body is mind, and this is the basis of psychosomatic philosophy.

References
Boss, M.: Existential Foundations of Medicine and Psychology. Jason Aronson; New Edition, 1995.
Heidegger, M., Boss, M., et al.: Zollikon Seminars Protocors-conversations-letters, Northwestern University Press. U.S. 2000.
von Weizsaecker, V.: Studien zur Pathogenese. Thieme, Wiesbaden 1946.

Heidegger, M.: Sein und Zeit, 1927.
Boss, M.: Psychoanalysis and Daseinsanalysis. Basic Books, 1963.
Boss, M.: The analyst of dream. Rider, 1957.
Kimura, B.: Zuwischen Mensch und Mensch. Wissenschaftliche Buchengesellschaft. Deutch, 2002.
Mizukami, E., Uesugi, T.: Imaging argument in Daseinsanalysis.Seishin-shobo, 1986.
Sartre, J. P.: 'the maxim of existentialism' from the methodology of the quest for truth, 1960.
Kimura, B.: Anthropology of Epilepsy. Tokyo Univ. publish. association, Tokyo, 1980.

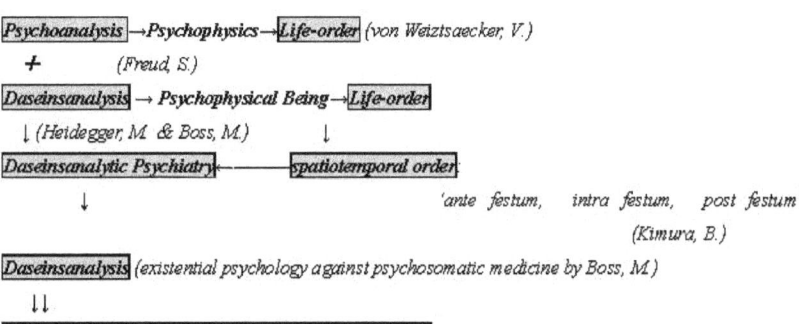

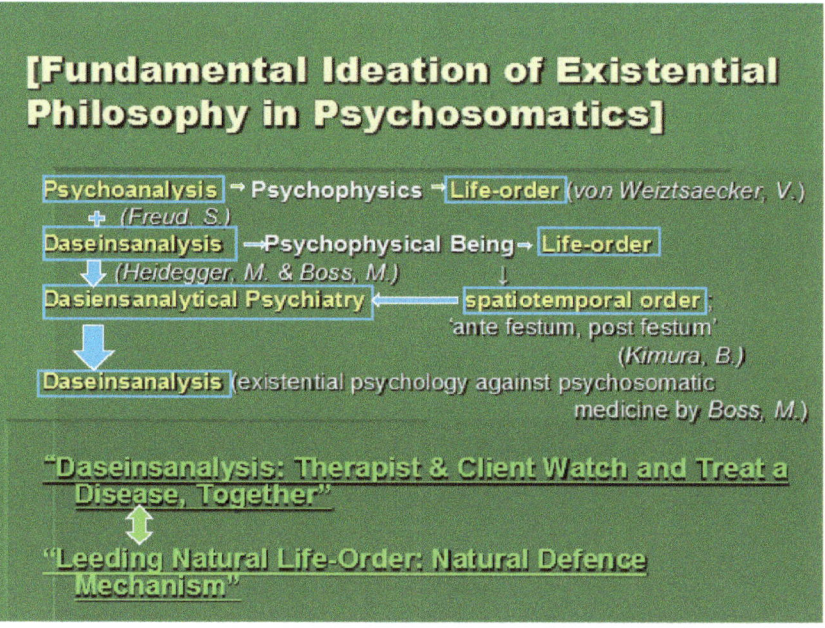

Figure 3. Fundamental Ideation of Existential Philosophy in Psychosomatics

Conclusion

In this philosophy, the human being is regarded as a Life-Order (Lebensordnung), and disease is identified as the crisis of that Life-Order (Lebensordnung Krise).

We can therefore conclude that when a human being suffers from disease, which is defined as the life-order crisis, he is still able to return to his natural life order with the help of Daseinsanalysis and SSRIs. In other words, Daseinsanalysis elevates immune responses in humans with the help of SSRIs.

PNIP demonstrates these phenomena practically and logically. With PNIP, any physician can treat any type of disease efficiently. PNIP will be particularly useful in the treatment of incurable diseases, so that the patients do not have to sit idly by and wait to die. PNIP exists for the sake of human beings who desire to live.

PNIP fundamentally differs from superficial treatments such as cognitive behavioral therapy and brief psychotherapy because PNIP is based on traditional psychopathology, which has been developing continuously for more than 100 years.

PNIP has been developed based on many fundamental experiments and experiences. Thus, PNIP was established by integrating neurology, immunology, psychopathology, and the important research areas of philosophy and evidence.

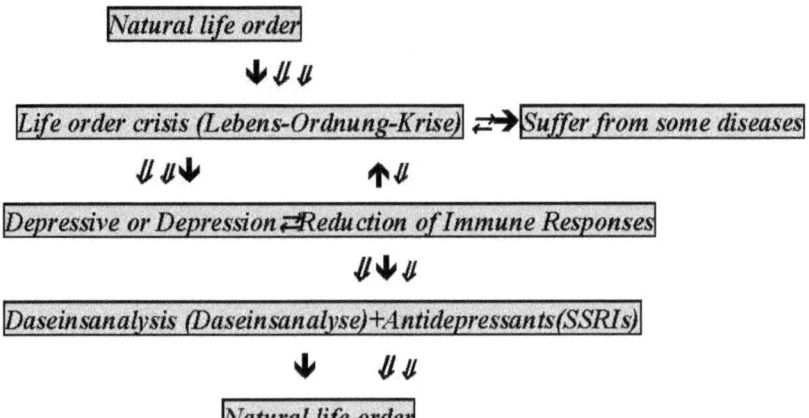

Figure 4: Human beings in Psychoneuroimmunopathology

Appendix

The author's daughter has a pet ferret. This ferret gradually showed abdominal swelling and was in pain. She consulted the author about whether the ferret had an abdominal disease. As soon as the author palpated the abdomen, he suspected that the ferret had a malignant tumor. She immediately took her ferret to a veterinarian for X-rays. She was informed by the veterinarian, "A big malignant tumor is visible in the abdomen in the X-rays. If you think an operation can remove the tumor, I will try, but I am not sure whether the operation will be successful or not. In any case, this ferret will die within two or three weeks, even if the operation is successful. If you do not do the operation, the ferret will die in several days."

She chose a third method, which was PNIP. She immediately went to the author and said, "Teach me PNIP and prescribe SSRIs. I will try PNIP for my ferret." The author answered, "Really?" because the author felt that it would be impossible for her to master PNIP. Fortunately, she completely mastered the techniques of PNIP used to treat human beings. However, instead of treating a human being, she wanted to treat a ferret, which had to be treated without using words. She tried PNIP repeatedly, accompanied by Fluvoxamine at a dose of 40 mg/day.

The ferret is alive, and the tumor has gotten smaller and smaller during the past month. Currently, only a small tumor is palpable in the ferret's abdomen. The ferret appears to actively enjoy playing with its partner and taking good long naps.

The author does not know how his daughter treated the ferret or what type of PNIP was used. Most likely, because the ferret's brain is simple, it might be recovering by simply from providing eu-stress and removing stressors. In any case, the ferret is actually making great progress toward recovery, similar to a human being.

Scientific experiments are usually performed on animals first, and then, when it is clear that the results are significant, the experiment is attempted on humans. However, the author believes that true medical science and treatment must be usable for any being on earth. This experience with the ferret validates the truth of this fundamental philosophy.

"Psychoneuroimmunopathology is clearly the most important area of research in theory and practice. The studies of PNIP will continue forever."

Index

Index
A
allergic reaction
aneurysm
ante festum
antidepressant
analytic
analysis
alpha wave
atopic dermatitis
attack
anxiety
asthma
Atypishe Psychose
B
Bence-Jones protein
bipolar disorder
C
carbamazepine
carcinoma
CD4
CD8

comrade
cognitive behavior therapy
catharsis
corticosteroid
cortisol
coronary heart disease
crisis
cytokine
cytolytic
cytotoxicity
D
dehydroepiandrosterone (DHEA)
depression
Diazepam
E
existential philosophy
enemy
F
ferret
Fluvoxamine
G
Glycyrrhizinic acid
H
Harrison method
hepato-cellular
I
IgE
IgG
IgM
IL-2
irritable bowel syndrome
immunoglobulin
immunology
intra festum
J

K
Krise

L
laughter training
Leader
Lebens
life history
life style
life-order

M
malignant
mind
Mirnacipran
myeloma

N
natural killer cell
neuroendocrinology
neoplasm

O
Ordnung

P
Paroxetine
phenomenology
post festum
psychopathology
psychoneuroimmunology (PNI)
psychophysics
psychosis
psychosomatic

Q

R
rape
RAST (radioallergosorbent test)
RIST (radioimmunosorbent test)

Rorschach test
S
schizoaffective disorder
seesaw phenomenon
severe depression
spatiotemporal
SNRI
spirit
SSRI
Stress Theory
T
T cell
terminal stage
T lymphocyte
Type A behavior
Type B behavior
U

V
Virchow lymph node
W

X

Y

Z

The author believes all human beings will be able to exist on earth only if their fundamental bio-psycho-socio-ethical existence is identified and acknowledged.

November 9, 2015

www.ingramcontent.com/pod-product-compliance
Lightning Source LLC
Chambersburg PA
CBHW040108180526
45172CB00009B/1268